MATERNAL DISTRESS
AND POSTNATAL DEPRESSION
The Myth of Madonna

LIBR

bc
r

MATERNAL DISTRESS AND POSTNATAL DEPRESSION

The Myth of Madonna

Jane Littlewood

Senior Lecturer in Social Policy and Politics
Goldsmiths' College, University of London

Nessa McHugh

Lecturer in Midwifery
De Montfort University, Leicester

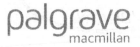

palgrave
macmillan

Published by
PALGRAVE MACMILLAN
Houndmills, Basingstoke, Hampshire RG21 6XS and
175 Fifth Avenue, New York, N. Y. 10010
Companies and representatives throughout the world

PALGRAVE MACMILLAN is the global academic imprint of the Palgrave Macmillan division of St. Martin's Press, LLC and of Palgrave Macmillan Ltd. Macmillan® is a registered trademark in the United States, United Kingdom and other countries. Palgrave is a registered trademark in the European Union and other countries.

ISBN 0–333–63834–4

This book is printed on paper suitable for recycling and made from fully managed and sustained forest sources.

A catalogue record for this book is available from the British Library.

10   9   8   7   6   5   4   3   2
11   10   09   08   07   06   05   04   03

Printed and bound in Great Britain by
Antony Rowe Ltd, Chippenham and Eastbourne

For Olive and Vivian

Written in the understanding that birth, like death, is a process that should not, in ordinary circumstances, be minimised, denied, manipulated or controlled.

Contents

List of Tables and Figures

Tables

Figures

Acknowledgements

This book initially grew out of research concerned with postnatal depression, stillbirth and neonatal death. Many discussions were held by a group of researchers concerned with Women and Welfare at Goldsmiths College, University of London. We would like to thank the group for their interest, their contributions and their patience. Many women who had suffered from postnatal depression were also kind enough to agree to contribute. We would like to thank them all for their honesty and their courage in speaking openly about an extremely painful experience. We hope that they will feel fairly represented by what is written here and that their experiences will be better understood.

This work has also benefited greatly from the many other researchers who have written about this area in an attempt to promote a more open discussion of women's experiences of postnatal depression. We would like to thank them all.

We owe particular thanks to Lesley Taylor for her support and her valuable work concerning the experiences of women who have given birth preterm. We also owe thanks to Carole Walker and Vivian Dhaliwal: to Carole for her support and practical assistance, and to Vivian for her valuable contributions and secretarial support.

Jane Littlewood would also like to thank Malcolm Nicholas for his resolute support and his valuable comments upon earlier versions of this manuscript.

Every effort has been made to trace all the copyright holders but, if any have been inadvertently overlooked, the publishers will be pleased to make the necessary arrangement at the first opportunity.

Introduction

This book is concerned with maternal distress and postnatal depression. It is about the ways in which women experience maternal distress and depression and the ways in which distress and depression are conceptualised by others. Consequently, Part I of the book introduces the major explanatory frameworks that have been developed in order better to understand postnatal depression and maternal distress.

Chapter 1 adopts a historical perspective upon social and cultural attitudes towards pregnancy and childbirth in general. Until relatively recently, childbirth was a hazardous transition that could, and frequently did, result in maternal death or debility. The religious discourses that associated distress with demonic possession, and pain during labour with maternal salvation, will be considered here. The growing dominance of medical discourses and the medicalisation of pregnancy and childbirth are also discussed. The decline in maternal and infant mortality, together with the growing recognition of postnatal depression as a distressing condition in its own right, is also documented in Chapter 1. The chapter concludes with a brief discussion of definitions of postnatal depression, estimates of incidence and major forms of screening and relevant treatment.

Chapter 2 commences with a consideration of organic models associated with the development of postnatal depression. Katharina Dalton's contribution to the area is assessed here. The chapter also reviews evidence associated with events occurring at, or around the time of, birth. Consequently, the association between the pathologisation of pregnancy, high levels of clinical intervention and maternal experiences of depression and/or distress are discussed in Chapter 2. The relevance of the clinical diagnosis of post-traumatic stress disorder to childbirth is documented alongside the related concept of birth trauma. The chapter concludes with an account of recent attempts to develop relevant models that are specific to trauma following childbirth.

Chapter 3 is concerned with the various psychological perspectives concerning maternal distress and postnatal depression. The chapter commences with a consideration of psychodynamic

1

approaches to the area. The second part of chapter three addresses issues raised by attachment theory, together with both lay and scientific 'theories' of mother–infant bonding. The chapter concludes with a discussion of cognitive approaches towards distress and depression following childbirth.

Chapter 4 identifies the various social and contextual explanations of maternal distress and depression. The first part of the chapter considers the relatively recent evidence that suggests that maternal distress and discomfort during the last trimester of pregnancy and the early postnatal period are almost universal experiences. The second part of the chapter is concerned with the relationship between various additional burdens of care falling upon the mother and the development of distress and/or depression. The third part of the chapter considers evidence associating maternity with loss. Loss of identity, self-esteem and role loss are all considered here. The chapter concludes with a discussion of the relationship between depression and oppression.

The second part of the book is concerned with women's experiences of postnatal depression and distress. Consequently, Chapter 5 adopts a broad sociocultural approach and investigates the ways in which the transition to motherhood is negotiated in other cultures. The second part of the chapter considers the concept of a 'rite of passage' and elements of ritualistic practice in Western societies. The final part of the chapter is concerned with the relationship between essentially unachievable cultural definitions of what it is to be a 'mother' and the development of postnatal depression and/or maternal distress.

Chapter 6 is directly concerned with motherhood and the experience of postnatal depression. The first part of the chapter addresses the issue of whether or not postnatal depression should be treated as a discrete psychiatric condition. The second part of the chapter is concerned with the experiences of five women who developed depression following the birth of their healthy children. The potential impact of physical birth trauma, psychological birth trauma, the reactivation of previous negative life experiences, the impact of inadequate social support networks and the loss of self-identify are all documented here.

Chapter 7 is concerned with motherhood, loss and distress. The first part of the chapter looks at the experience of women who give birth preterm and who are separated from their babies shortly after the birth has occurred. The chapter also considers the additional burdens of care throughout pregnancy and after birth for women

2

who become the mothers of more than one baby. The impact of the birth of a mentally and/or physically impaired baby is discussed, as is the often long-term distress and disruption associated with 'voluntarily' relinquishing a baby for fostering or adoption. The multiple losses experienced by women who are HIV-positive or have the AIDS syndrome are identified, and the chapter concludes with a consideration of a generic model of coping when motherhood is 'uncertain'.

Chapter 8 documents the range of experiences that mothers undergo when a baby dies at, or around the time of, birth. The range of experiences associated with miscarriage and abortion are discussed in this chapter. Maternal distress associated with expected and unexpected stillbirths and neonatal deaths are also considered here. The unique problems associated with the death of a twin leaving a surviving infant are identified, and the chapter concludes with a discussion concerning the impact the death of a baby may have upon the future childbearing of the mother.

The final chapter is concerned with the range of support available once distress and/or depression are established. Consequently, a broad range of self-help initiatives is identified and evaluated. The value of the Edinburgh Postnatal Depression Scale as a screening device is identified and the distinct lack of resources, coupled with the absence of geographical equity, discussed. Unfortunately, a marked lack of reporting distress and depression associated with fear of being perceived as a 'bad' and/or 'inadequate' mother is also identified. Perhaps the 'myth of Madonna' has a great deal to answer for; until we all refrain from subscribing to a series of sociocultural myths concerning motherhood, postnatal depression and maternal distress will continue to blight what could be, and should be, an exciting and exhilarating time during which a woman gets to know her new baby.

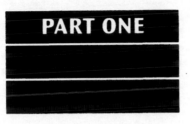

PART ONE

MODELS OF MATERNAL DISTRESS AND POSTNATAL DEPRESSION

Chapter 1

Maternity and Madness

Indeed, childbirth was seen by some religious thinkers as 'woman's hour of sorrow' when, in conditions of 'peculiar agony' each mother would reflect upon the fall and experience her pain as 'a lasting memorial' of Eve's fate and 'an impressive comment on the evil nature of sin'.

(Davidoff and Hall, 1987, p. 114)

It is difficult to consider postnatal depression without looking at social and cultural attitudes towards pregnancy and childbirth in general. Whilst maternal mortality is now relatively rare and the vast majority of women who wish to deliver a live baby safely will do so, postnatal depression and maternal distress remain problems that affect a significant proportion of mothers. Historically, childbirth was once a hazardous transition that not infrequently resulted in death or debility for women, and the very real dangers involved must have affected women's perceptions of their experiences. Also, the limited availability at this time of reliable contraception often led to closely spaced births, numerous children and general maternal debilitation (Davidoff and Hall, 1987). In addition, 'madness' has long been associated with femininity in general, if not with maternity in particular. Consequently, the first part of this chapter looks at some of the ways in which these issues may have clouded our historical perspective.

The second part of this chapter focuses primarily upon the inter-war period in Britain. It was at this time that pregnancy and childbirth started to become a medical (and arguably 'masculine') concern rather than a communal (and arguably 'feminine') one. It was also during this period that mental disturbance following childbirth was acknowledged in law by the passing of the 1932 Infanticide Act.

The third part of the chapter looks at some of the evidence suggesting that the medicalisation of pregnancy and childbirth, which accelerated during the latter part of the twentieth century, has, coupled with other changes in social policy, paradoxically resulted in an increase in the number of women likely to suffer from postnatal depression. The potential impact of recent policy changes following the Winterton Report will also be considered here.

The final part of the chapter will be concerned with our contemporary understanding and definitions of postnatal depression and maternal distress. Problems associated with the measurement, evaluation and treatment of postnatal depression and maternal distress will conclude the chapter.

Maternity, demonic possession and madness

One of the first references to psychological and/or physiological disturbances following childbirth was made by Hippocrates (cited in Lloyd, 1978). Specifically, Hippocrates commented upon the development of what he called 'milk fever'. Hippocrates was of the opinion that, in certain unspecified circumstances, milk fever could occur at the onset of lactation (about 3–4 days postpartum). This 'fever' was associated with physical and psychological symptoms that included episodes of weeping and hysteria. Whilst it may be tempting, in the contemporary situation, to account for these observations in terms of an early account of postnatal 'blues', they could equally well be associated with the onset of puerperal infection.

Relatively few other references seem to have been made concerning psychological disturbances following childbirth until the Middle Ages. Again, what has been written in this context is difficult to interpret owing to the unknown prevalence of puerperal infection. However, difficulties also arise from an association between mental disturbance and possession by demons. For example, one of the earliest surviving English autobiographies, that of the anchoress Margery Kempe, gives a poignant insight into the concerns of women during the period. Margery begins her account of her life with the 'spiritual crisis' she experienced following the birth of her first child. Whilst this crisis was eventually resolved after Margery saw the vision of Christ, which stimulated her religious learning, her description of her experience is harrowing:

> Therefore, after her child was born, and not believing she would live, ...this creature went out of her mind and was amazingly disturbed and tormented with spirits for half a year, eight weeks and odd days.
>
> *(Kempe, 1989, p. 41)*

Margery's fears were concerned not only with the distinct possibility of death, but also with the certainty of damnation. During the

8

time that Margery was 'out of her mind', she experienced visual and auditory hallucinations in which demons from hell tempted and clawed at her in order to make her speak 'out of character'. Margery slandered her husband, her friends and herself, and experienced severe suicidal impulses that led to several attempts at self-harm:

> She would have killed herself many a time as they stirred her to... and it is witness of this she bit her own hand so violently that the mark could be seen for the rest of her life. And also she pitilessly tore the skin on her body with her nails... and she would have done something far worse except that she was tied up and forcibly restrained both day and night so that she could not do as she wanted.
>
> *(Kempe, 1989, p. 42)*

It is impossible to say whether Margery's condition was a result of extreme fear followed by puerperal infection or of a combination of other factors. Nevertheless, her description of being caught between:

> the dread of damnation on the one hand... and his [her confessor's] sharp reproving of her on the other
>
> *(Kempe, 1989, p. 41)*

vividly illustrates the perceptions of a woman who, legitimately or otherwise, felt she had nowhere and no-one to turn to.

Outside Margery Kempe's description of being 'out of her mind' following childbirth, there were many factors prevalent in the Middle Ages that would have effectively masked any widespread documentation of distress following childbirth, specifically:

- High maternal and child mortality rates;
- An emphasis upon the life-or-death nature of childbirth;
- An interpretation of intense physical pain and psychological suffering within a religious framework that presumed women to be responsible for original sin;
- Relatively poor physical health coupled with a focus on day-to-day survival that did not necessarily include any notions of psychological wellbeing.

In short, psychological distress may have either gone unacknowledged or, if it resulted in severely disturbed behaviour, have been taken as evidence of demonic possession. Owing to the widespread acceptance of the ideology of the Church, the medical knowledge that was available at the time was in the hands of men, but childbirth was considered to be an unsuitable area for male involvement. Consequently, childbirth became the domain of women who, since they were not allowed into the medical schools, had no formal training. Furthermore, what was considered to be 'medical' knowledge at the time was concerned with physical rather than mental or spiritual matters. These matters would have fallen outside the sphere of medicine but within the sphere of the Church.

Paradoxically, women's involvement in assisting childbirth was viewed with intense suspicion by both the Church and the medical profession. Women in general were believed to be weakened by the burden of original sin and were thus likely to become the prime suspects if demonic influences were either implicated or detected. Thus, the *Malleus Malificarum* (1486) specifically identified midwives, a group of women who out of necessity operated outside the dominant sphere of male control, as prime suspects of witchcraft. Therefore, it would seem probable that maternal distress, if it became evident, would be interpreted in terms of sin and/or demonic possession rather than illness or psychological distress.

Unfortunately, when mental disorder rather than demonic possession began to be recognised in its own right, women fared little better. As early as the seventeenth century, the files of a Dr R. Napier (1981) indicated that nearly twice as many cases of mental disorder could be found amongst his female patients when compared with his male patients, and as Showalter (1987) has indicated, women by the 1850s formed the majority of the asylum inmate population. Nevertheless, up until this time there was little real recognition of mental trauma, aside from reminders of 'sin', which were associated with childbirth in particular rather than women in general.

However, by the eighteenth century the Church's position concerning the 'necessity' of the social and spiritual subordination of women had changed somewhat. Whilst women were still held to be socially subordinate, their very subordination became equated with their salvation. Women, by following the social path of domesticity and maternity could redeem themselves in order to achieve the necessary spiritual equality equated with salvation. For example:

> But childbirth could also represent a woman's access to salvation since Mary, the mother of Jesus, had through her maternity raised woman from despair. Christian notions of womanhood thus assumed a link between the godly woman and her family duties.
>
> *(Davidoff and Hall, 1987, p. 114)*

Given the prevalent ideology at the time, it would surely be unthinkable to respond to one's salvation by admitting depression rather than euphoria following the birth of a child. Furthermore, if such a situation arose, it would appear likely that attempts would be made to manage the problem in private rather than to seek help in public.

Charlotte Perkins Gilman (1981) wrote a fictional account of what is now widely regarded to be postnatal depression. Gilman herself suffered from depression, and *The Yellow Wallpaper* draws on her own experiences and treatment. The woman in the story (she is never named) is totally isolated by her doctor husband from family and friends and is made to take a complete 'rest cure'. She is not allowed to read, write or sew, and she is not allowed to look after her own child. The woman's depressive behaviour was, arguably, treated as a threat to the prevailing cultural ideology of the time, and she was consequently removed from the public sphere. Gilman's work shows the extent to which male control determined an appropriate therapy to produce the desired behaviour associated with the 'angel in the home' ideology. For the woman in *The Yellow Wallpaper*, it is only in her madness that she can escape the constraints placed upon her by society.

Alternatively, Showalter (1988) has argued that, if sensitively applied, and given the prevailing ideology of the time we can only presume that this would have been a relatively rare occurrence, the rest cure could be used to liberate women from the debilitating ideal of angelic womanhood. Specifically:

> The rest cure made women who were denying their bodies, their appetites, and their sensations confront nothing but the body, the appetite, and the senses for a prolonged period. This cannot have been entirely a bad thing.
>
> *(Showalter, 1987, p. 140)*

Showalter also indicates that many women who were subjected to the rest cure were:

> women reacting to traumatic miscarriages, stillbirths of painful deliveries that had left them physically and emotionally scarred. In case after case, their immobility, sensitivity, loss of appetite, and depression seem to be forms of sexual withdrawal, the body protecting itself against further invasion.
>
> *(Showalter, 1987, p. 140)*

However, it was not until the middle of the nineteenth century that the predominantly religious discourses regarding the problems women experienced following childbirth were thoroughly overtaken by the rapidly developing medical discourses concerning both physical disease and mental disorder. In 1858 a Parisian doctor, Dr Marcé, was of the opinion that previously emotionally stable women could be prone to episodes of instability associated with the birth of their child. He divided his observations into those associated with women who suffered from immediate puerperal illnesses and those associated with women for whom the onset of symptoms developed within 6 weeks postpartum.

Contemporary medical opinion differs concerning the significance of Marcé's original findings. In particular, it has been argued that the symptoms he observed and recorded could also be found in other forms of mental illness. Alternatively, Hamilton (1989) considered that Marcé had made a significant contribution in distinguishing between mental illnesses in general and puerperal cases in particular. However, the issues are almost certainly complicated by the lack of availability of effective antibiotic treatment at the time of Marcé's observations. Any interpretation concerning the contribution of Marcé must accommodate the relatively common occurrence of confusional psychoses secondary to major infections. Solomons (1931) argued that toxaemia and sepsis were amongst the most common causes of puerperal psychosis (not to mention maternal mortality). Hemphill (1952) also followed this line of argument by suggesting that the total number of psychoses in the puerperium had decreased over the years more or less directly in line with the availability of antibiotics that effectively controlled the toxic conditions.

However, the situation was further complicated by maternal fear of death. For example, the following comments were made by a working class woman in England in 1914:

I always prepared myself to die, and I think this awful depression is common to most at this time.
                                                                (cited in Shorter, 1991, p. 70)

Whilst Marcé's observations are clearly open to qualification, perhaps their true significance lies in their recognition of mental distress associated with childbirth. However, this recognition was deemed, at least in Britain, to be of less significance than the health and wellbeing of babies. Concern over the health of the population in Britain was stimulated by the poor physical condition of recruits for the Boer War. This concern led to the establishment of various committees and Acts of Parliament (Table 1.1). Despite the fact that the majority of reports and subsequent legislation focused upon the health of children, women eventually benefited, at least initially, from increased and increasing state concern and intervention in the processes of childbearing and rearing.

Table 1.1 Response to concerns over poor health

1902	Midwives Act
1904	Interdepartmental Committee on Physical Deterioration set up
1907	Notification of Births Act passed
1918	Maternity and Child Welfare Act passed

Source: Ham 1984.

The 1902 Midwives Act established a split between the functions associated with laying out the dead and attending the birth of babies. Most women opted to concentrate upon midwifery, and this act eventually led to a decline in female 'layers out'. This decline preceded a rise in the still largely masculine occupations of funeral director and embalmer (Gore, 1995). The 1902 Act also established the principle of the Registry of midwives.

The 1904 Interdepartmental Committee on Physical Deterioration paved the way for the school medical service and free school meals. The 1907 Notification of Births Act was particularly influential. As Ham indicates:

> The 1907 Act helped the development of health visiting by enabling local authorities to insist on the compulsory notification of births. An Act of 1915 placed a duty on local authorities to ensure compulsory notification.
>
> *(Ham, 1984, p. 10)*

The 1918 Maternity and Child Welfare Act introduced family allowances and the maternity grant. In short, the state strongly registered its interest in the health and wellbeing of babies. Following World War I, this interest was further consolidated by various measures that occurred during the inter-war period.

Inter-war Britain

Whilst the early years of the twentieth century were marked by an increase in concern over the social and physical wellbeing of mothers, concern over their psychological health was not as marked. However, the experience of childbirth and childbearing, given the lack of widespread availability of contraception, could still be a harrowing one. For example:

Many a time I have sat in daddy's big chair, a baby $2^1/_2$ years old at my back, one 16 months and one 1 month on my knees and cried for very weariness and hopelessness.

(Llewelyn-Davies, 1915, p. 45)

and

I have been most fortunate and have had very good times, so they tell me, but the best of times are bad enough.

(Llewelyn-Davies, 1915, p. 91)

As Oakley (1979) has indicated, the social and medical management of childbirth and childcare was, from the end of the nineteenth century, changing from a structure of control located in a community of formally untrained women to one based upon formally trained health-care professionals. The inter-war period saw an acceleration of this process as the state became more and more involved with the provision of care for mothers and babies.

The 1930s saw the increasing isolation of women in the community, together with the continuing development of theories concerning childrearing that maintained the centrality of the 'trained mother' for the success of the process. For example, as Liddiard (1923) has indicated Truby-King's ideas concerning mothercraft involved the setting of rigid routines for mothers and babies. These routines were overtly designed to secure physically and mentally healthy children and reflected earlier concerns relating to the lack of fitness of war recruits for the Boer War. The development of the almost militaristic childrearing regimes of the 1930s was a natural extension of these concerns. Truby-King believed that women had a 'maternal instinct' and wanted to care for children, but that they had no natural knowledge of how to socialise them. Maternal education was based upon a hygienist approach and little attention was given to the benefits of play and intimacy. Richardson has suggested that much of the childrearing literature of the 1930s actively contributed towards making mothering even more demanding because:

Mothers were now held responsible not only for the physical and moral welfare of their children, but also for their psychological development.

(Richardson, 1993, p. 37)

14

Richardson (1993) goes on to note that, as greater professional interest and concern over child development became institutionalised, this led to an increase in the social control and surveillance of women as mothers. Women could now realistically expect social disapproval, the possible removal of their child or prosecution if they were perceived to be failing to perform their new maternal 'duties' adequately. Childcare was rapidly becoming the province of, usually self-proclaimed, 'experts'.

Further interest in the physical 'fitness' of women to become mothers during the 1930s came with the Departmental Committee on Maternal Mortality and Morbidity in 1930 and 1932. The committee placed particular importance on the provision of adequate antenatal care, which led to an expansion of antenatal clinics and more expert intervention in childbirth. In addition, this committee's deliberations, followed by the 1936 Midwives Act, led to the development of a salaried midwifery service.

The 1930s also saw the passing of the 1932 Infanticide Act, which gave some formal recognition to the possibility of altered mental states following childbirth and lactation. The crime of infanticide was only available to women who were responsible for the death of their newly born babies (up to 1 year). This Act explicitly recognised that a woman could commit infanticide when 'at the time of the act or omission she had not fully recovered from the effect of lactation and for this reason the balance of her mind was disturbed'. Historically, the Act represented an improvement upon the harsh treatment previously meted out to mothers who killed their children, but with the benefit of hindsight and with contemporary knowledge concerning postnatal depression, it seems that women were being treated as human beings who were totally at the mercy of their biology and that the weakness identified in the fourteenth century, that is, a proneness to succumbing to demonic influence, had effectively been replaced in the former half of the twentieth century by the identification of an alternative weakness, that of succumbing to hormonal influence. The main provisions of the Infanticide Act were eventually incorporated in the 1957 Homicide Act. As Cameron and Frazer indicate, infanticide is said to occur:

Where a woman kills her child of less than one year because she is suffering from the effects of pregnancy or lactation. This is an offence men cannot commit (though they can kill infants and frequently do). The penalty tends to be light, since these women are seen as victims of their biology.

(Cameron and Frazer, 1987, p. 7)

Despite being incorporated into the Homicide Act, the Infanticide Act effectively remains on the statute book, and Kennedy succinctly identifies both the problematic nature of the situation together with a potential solution:

> Since the creation of the special female crime of infanticide, the law has come to a greater understanding of mental impairment. The 1957 Homicide Act created a special defence to murder, reducing it to manslaughter where the offender's criminal responsibility was diminished because of such impairment. The infanticide law involved a paternalistic and generalised approach to women's psychology and physiology, and it should be removed from the statute book and absorbed into the Homicide Act. Childbirth and lactation do not dissolve all women's brains, but severe postnatal depression is a recognised disorder and would fulfil the criteria for diminished responsibility in appropriate cases.
>
> *(Kennedy, 1992, p. 103)*

Paradoxically, it was only when the physical problems associated with childbirth were finally almost completely overcome by antibiotics and blood transfusions that postnatal depression began to be recognised as a problem in its own right. These developments took place alongside the increasing availability of effective contraception that enabled women to space births more effectively and to limit the size of their families. Equally paradoxically, the major forces behind these positive changes – the development of the National Health Service (NHS) and the professionalisation of those who cared for pregnant women – were the very forces charged with increasing the incidence of postnatal depression amongst the mothers of babies born after World War II.

The medicalisation of pregnancy and childbirth

Following World War II, the 'Beveridge blueprint' (an attempt to facilitate the creation of a society fit for heroes to live in) was actively promoted by the government of the day. The 'blueprint' was essentially an attempt at social engineering that involved exceptionally clear ideas regarding the social position of women who were firmly designated within the National Insurance and social security systems as the dependents of men. Marriage, in some cases under threat due to lengthy wartime separations, was also deemed to be an institution worthy of state support. The ideal position for any woman was seen to be that of somebody's wife and somebody's mother. Women who had previously been working to support the war effort were actively encouraged to give up paid work and return to their 'natural' position as homemakers. As is often the way with wars, World War II was followed by a 'baby boom'. For the new mothers of post-war Britain who were full-time childrearers and wives, their future was construed, primarily by men, to be bright indeed. For example, *The Motherhood Book* (1949), whose market was to be the expectant mother and whose scope was to cover the baby's first years, was compiled by 'a distinguished group of experts and specialists in health, maternity, infant and child welfare'. This book covers most aspects of pregnancy and childbirth, including factors governing the choice of whether to give birth at home or in a nursing home. The work even includes a chapter concerned with the special needs of preterm babies. What the work does not cover is any mention of the possibility of the onset of the 'baby blues' or of postnatal depression proper. Presumably, the Beveridge blueprint had done for mothers in the mid-twentieth century what Protestantism had done for them in the mid-nineteenth century: on the crest of a wave of ideological constructions of motherhood, maternal experiences of distress were presumed simply to have disappeared.

Further constraints were placed upon mothers by the publication of a series of papers by John Bowlby (for example, 1951), which strongly suggested that mother and child should stay in close proximity to each other and that maternal deprivation, even of a short duration, was associated with long-term deleterious psychological consequences for the child. Despite this work being challenged (for example, by Rutter, 1966), and modified, Bowlby's observations dovetailed nicely into the post-war state's policy preoccupations, and the work was highly influential in informing a social policy that encouraged mothers to stay at home in order to care for their preschool children. The impact of isolation upon mothers, given geographical mobility and, in some instances, the breakdown of communities following World War II, was not even considered to be problematic until the second wave of feminism in the 1960s. However, as Ussher so poignantly illustrates, this impact was apparently felt by at least one woman:

What I *do* know is that mother was not mad, and that her anger, pain and despair were not unique to her. I know that women trapped in unhappy marriages, isolated, lonely, with young, demanding children, no money and no friends are often deemed mad. That to be a woman is often to be mad. If we stay inside our prescribed roles and routes as my mother did, or if we speak out, or move outside out designated paths we become mad. My mother may have been mad because she was adhering to the dictates of her feminine role, staying as wife and mother when she desperately wanted to flee.

(Ussher, 1991, pp. 5–6)

However, by far the most important impact of post-war policy came from the development of the NHS and the incorporation of midwifery within it. Paradoxically, a policy innovation that was associated with an increase in safety, measured by a decrease in both maternal and infant mortality, has also been associated with an increase in the susceptibility of women to postnatal depression and distress. Postnatal depression was increasingly identified as a discrete condition in its own right.

As maternal mortality figures dropped due to the availability of antibiotics and blood transfusions, pregnancy and childbirth became increasingly controlled by the predominantly male medical profession, and the place of birth moved from either at home or in a nursing home, to the hospital. This shift in location rapidly accelerated following World War II. As Chamberlain indicates:

> Until the mid-1930s maternal mortality was the same as it had been in Victorian times. With the development of chemotherapy and antibiotics the rates reduced; to this was added the improvements brought by a proper blood transfusion service catalysed by the second world war. The founding of the colleges of obstetrics (1929) and midwives (1933) organised professional training and standards, and the unification of the antenatal and delivery services in the new NHS helped further.
>
> *(Chamberlain, 1991, p. 477)*

Consequently, by the 1960s the Peel Report (1970) was calling for 100 per cent hospital confinements for pregnant women. This call was echoed by the Court Report in 1976, and Welburn (1980), amongst others, has suggested that the medicalisation of childbirth, together with the associated disempowerment of women, is enough in itself to be implicated as a cause of postnatal distress and depression. She cites births that are associated with high levels of medical intervention as presenting particular problems for women. For example:

> It is not uncommon for caesarean operations to be performed because an induction fails. What this woman's story clearly indicates is that *she* connects a long postnatal depression directly with a bad birth experience which she feels was a doctor created emergency. She wanted to give birth naturally and has lost that experience. Her labour had been artificially controlled throughout.
>
> *(Welburn, 1980, p. 94)*

The increasing isolation of the labouring woman from both familiar surroundings and people has also been cited as exacerbating maternal distress. As Mead has indicated:

No primitive society leaves the mother alone, nor does any leave her alone among strangers

(Mead, 1971, p. 21)

Kitzinger (1992) has argued that many women become depressed after 'birth trauma' that is associated with a disregard of the mother as a person coupled with a focus upon the 'medical production' of a live baby. Women typically report being treated 'like a piece of meat' and are understandably traumatised by such treatment. Whilst the Winterton Report (1992) has done much to recognise and address these problems, whether or not the report will result in effective policy changes remains to be seen. Certainly, the focus upon women being 'active partners' in pregnancy and childbirth is to be encouraged, but the disparity in power between the pregnant or labouring woman and the various health-care professionals with whom she comes into contact is likely to remain a real one. The indicators of the success in *Changing Childbirth* are given in Appendix I.

Our contemporary understanding of postnatal depression

Whilst the bulk of the literature pertaining to postnatal depression has been written in the past 40 years, maternal distress has rarely been considered. Furthermore, most standard textbooks for midwives, nurses, obstetricians and psychiatrists still make scant reference to postnatal depression.

Possibly the most readily recognised definition of postnatal depression has been supplied by Dalton (1980). Dalton defines postnatal depression as the first psychiatric illness occurring within the first 6 months after childbirth that requires medical intervention. In addition to this, Dalton has broken down the general term 'postnatal depression' to give a more precise idea of the psychological disturbances that are involved. These disturbances are considered, by Dalton, to be interrelated but potentially separate conditions. The first type of disturbance is that of the postpartum blues, which commonly occurs around the third day postpartum. It is assumed that postpartum blues are a result of fluctuating hormone levels that result from the expulsion of the placenta in the third stage of labour and the establishment of lactation around the third day postpartum. Dalton further identifies the psychological disturbances and severe physical exhaustion that may result in moderate-to-severe postnatal depression. This can occur as a gradual onset from postpartum blues and can manifest itself at any point up to approximately 6 months postpartum.

The final disturbance identified is that of puerperal psychosis. In this instance, the onset is usually sudden and within a few days postpartum. Puerperal psychosis is typically characterised by severe behavioural changes and psychotic episodes. Women affected by puerperal psychosis may experience auditory and visual hallucinations. This form of psychological disturbance probably has the highest detection rate owing to the severe nature of its manifestation, which typically occurs whilst the woman is still undergoing a period of hospitalisation. The postpartum blues are also potentially easy to detect for similar reasons. However, postnatal depression may present problems because of (a) the nature of onset and, perhaps more importantly, (b) a social construction of motherhood that renders depression 'unspeakable' and therefore something to be hidden, if possible, from health-care workers who may be able to help.

The symptoms associated with the above cited disturbances are described below.

Postpartum blues

Symptoms include bursting into tears for no apparent reason, various anxieties (for example, inability to cope), fatigue, associated difficulty in sleeping and poor appetite. Negative emotional experiences are believed to peak at around the fifth day postpartum (Kendell *et al.*, 1984). Postpartum blues are not usually considered to be a psychiatric condition and may often be a fleeting phenomenon.

Moderate-to-severe depressive disorder

Symptoms include various anxieties, tearfulness, confusion, inappropriate obsessional thoughts, irritability, confusion, fatigue, insomnia, guilt, fear of harming the baby and loss of interest in sexual activity. Some women also report personality changes (for example, becoming unusually irritable and/or angry with members of their family). According to Gilbert (1992), these personality changes may add to the woman's sense of loss and further reduce her self-esteem. The impact of a moderate-to-severe depressive disorder following childbirth has been found to be long lasting. For example, Cox *et al.*, (1984) found that at least half of the mothers in their sample had not recovered after 1 year. Also, it has been found that other problems, for example agoraphobia, may date from the onset of a depressive episode, and evidence suggests that these problems are not short lived but may continue for months or even years (O'Hara and Zekoski, 1988).

Puerperal psychosis

Puerperal psychosis is comparatively rare, the majority of cases being classified as affective illnesses (Platz and Kendell, 1988). Puerperal psychosis requires inpatient hospital treatment.

Perhaps unsurprisingly, the literature concerning the statistical occurrence of postnatal depression is conflicting owing to difficulties associated with detection. For example, the Marcé Society (1980) put the incidence as follows:

Postpartum blues	8 in 10 women
Moderate/severe depression	2 in 10 women
Puerperal psychosis	2 in 3 000 women

However, other estimates are readily available in the literature. For example, Yalom et al. (1968) have argued that the rate of postpartum blues is so high that this condition should be anticipated as a normal part of childbirth. Furthermore, Paykel (1980) has argued that women who develop postnatal depression have an underlying disposition that inclines them towards depression and that on these grounds postnatal depression should not be seen as a psychiatric condition in its own right. However, other research would strongly suggest that postnatal depression is a condition specific to childbirth and that the women who are affected do not necessarily have any underlying personality traits that may act as triggers (Baker, 1967). Furthermore, Dalton's (1980) definition actively excludes women who have previously been treated for a prior psychiatric condition. However, it must be said that many women experience psychological distress and that they be unable or unwilling to report this owing to the stigma associated with mental illness. As Gilbert (1992) indicates, recent media coverage has brought about public awareness of postnatal depression as a distressing condition that goes unrecognised by physicians and health-care professionals. Cox et al. (1982) found that 13 out of the 101 women they interviewed had a marked depressive illness, the majority of which had gone untreated despite visits from health visitors and GP awareness of the patient's state.

In summary, postnatal depression has proven both difficult to detect and difficult to measure. It is questionable whether standard measuring instruments (for example, the Beck Depression Inventory) are appropriate. Some researchers (Cox et al., 1987) have devised special screening measures (The Edinburgh Postnatal Depression Scale; see Appendix II) but Cox et al. (1987) point out that self-report schedules are not alternatives for proper clinical assessments and that some cases of postnatal depression may not conform to standard descriptions.

Also, there are many different types of treatment and routes of referral in the case of postnatal depression. For example, referrals may be made by a midwife or health visitor to a doctor, a psychiatrist, a psychiatric nurse or a community psychiatric nurse. Assessment is usually carried out by interview, sometimes accompanied by the use of relevant diagnostic questionnaires.

Treatment may involve a combination of different interventions. Antidepressants, of which there are a number of different types, are sometimes the only form of treatment. In certain instances, interactive therapies may be used. For example, generic counselling or specific therapeutic interventions may also be recommended (such as cognitive therapy), accompanied by medication if this is seen to be appropriate. Counselling can come from any number of sources, depending upon local resources: trained health visitors, GPs or community psychiatric nurses. Other sources include voluntary or charitable organisations, including the Samaritans, local voluntary counselling services, the National Childbirth Trust, 'Meet-a-Mum', the Society for Postnatal Illness and Homestart (see Appendix IV for more information on these organisations). Psychotherapy is also available in some areas.

Some women will be admitted to hospital where treatment may take the form of electro-convulsive therapy (ECT) in instances of severe depression. Medication and other therapeutic support may also be offered. Facilities vary on a regional basis, some health authorities providing special mother and baby units and others providing for admission of mother and baby to generic psychiatric wards. Hospital treatment is also available on both an *ad hoc* and an outpatient basis. In addition, progesterone therapy is also available from some GPs. This usually consists of a series of progesterone injections, suppositories and tablets, which are believed to act as prophylactic therapy for women deemed to be at risk of developing postnatal depression.

Conclusion

The early historical references to postnatal distress, whilst moving, are relatively rare and extremely difficult to isolate from the prevalent ideology at the relevant time. Hippocrates may have observed, but did not comment upon, the psychological implication for the mother of 'milk fever', and references from the Middle Ages tend to be obscured by beliefs concerning demonic possession. For example, hallucinations were commonly thought to be caused by demonic possession and/or malevolent curses. Furthermore, the role played by potential physical causes of postpartum psychological changes and the fear, not to mention the very real possibility, of maternal death only add to a confused and confusing picture.

The rise of Protestantism and the equating of motherhood with salvation from original sin also added to the already considerable ambiguity by rendering the discussion of postpartum distress socially difficult. Furthermore, the increasing professionalisation of notions concerning child development and the ever-increasing level of state intervention following concern over the health of army recruits must have added to maternal anxieties surrounding the importance of being perceived to be a good mother. Even in the earlier part of the twentieth century, it seems reasonable to suggest that postnatal distress was an under-reported phenomenon.

Lack of widespread availability of contraception, coupled with relatively high rates of maternal mortality, further confused the picture associated with the inter-war years in Britain. Whilst the inter-war years saw one of the first formal indicators of maternal distress following childbirth (the Infanticide Act), multiple, closely spaced births, coupled with general fatigue, made the incidence of postnatal distress, apart from that which resulted in murder, difficult to determine.

The period that followed World War II and the associated medicalisation and hospitalisation of childbirth were associated with problems of their own. The marginalisation of the pregnant and/or labouring mother from her own community has been associated with an increase in postnatal depression, as has the increasingly medical (and masculine) approach to childbirth. Furthermore, broader social policy initiatives have been implicated in contributing to the isolation and anxieties that many women experience following childbirth. These social policy initiatives may also have made it less, rather than more, likely that any woman will be willing to seek help for postpartum distress.

At the present time, postnatal depression would appear to be difficult to predict, measure and treat. The current situation is one in which mental illness is still a social stigma. In the case of postnatal depression, this stigma may be compounded by our cultural images of motherhood. Contemporary society still portrays the ability to mother as a naturally occurring and inherently 'feminine' quality. To suffer mental distress associated with motherhood is therefore 'unnatural', and society has traditionally and relentlessly condemned the unnatural woman/mother. The fear for many women is that their baby will be taken from them if they acknowledge the fact that they are experiencing such 'unnatural' distress.

Paradoxically, the medicalisation of childbirth, which has been widely criticised as contributing towards postnatal depression and maternal distress, has also done a great deal to bring the problem to public attention. There is an increasing amount of evidence suggesting that distressing events at, or around the time of, birth may result in postnatal depression and/or maternal distress. This evidence will be reviewed in Chapter 2.

References

Baker, A. A. (1967) *Psychiatric Disorders in Obstetrics* (Oxford: Blackwell Scientific).

Bowlby, J. (1951) *Maternal Care and Mental Health. WHO Monograph Series No. 2* (Geneva: WHO).

Cameron, D. and Frazer, E. (1987) *The Lust to Kill: A Feminist Investigation of Sexual Murder* (Cambridge: Polity Press).

Chamberlain, G. (1991) 'Vital Statistics of Birth.' *MIDIRS Midwifery Digest* 1(4): 475–8.

Court Report (1976) *Fit for the Future*. Report of the Committee on Child Health Services, Cmnd 6684 (London: HMSO).

Cox, J. L., Connor, Y. and Kendall, R. E. (1982) 'Prospective Study of the Psychiatric Disorders of Childbirth.' *British Journal of Psychiatry* **140**: 11–117.

Cox, J. L., Rooney, A., Thomas, A. and Wrate, R. M. (1984) 'How Accurately Do Mothers Recall Postnatal Depression?' *Journal of Psychosomatic Obstetrics and Gynaecology* **3**: 185–7.

Cox, J. L., Holden, J. M. and Sagovsky, R. (1987) 'Detection of Postnatal Depression: development of the Edinburgh Postnatal Depression Scale.' *British Journal of Psychiatry* **130**: 782–8.

Dalton, K. (1980) *Depression After Childbirth* (Oxford: Open University Press).

Davidoff, L. and Hall, C. (1987) *Family Fortunes – Men and Women of the English Middle Class* (London: Hutchinson).

Gilbert, P. (1992) *Depression: the Evolution of Powerlessness* (Hove: Lawrence Erlbaum Associates).

Gilman, C. P. (1981) *The Yellow Wallpaper and Other Fiction* (London: Woman's Press).

Gore, P. (1995) 'The Funeral Industry: Embalmers and Embalming'. Unpublished paper presented to the 2nd International Conference on The Social Context of Death and Dying, University of Sussex, 17 September.

Ham, C. (1984) *Health Policy in Britain*, 2nd edn (London: Macmillan).

Hamilton, J. A. (1989) 'Postpartum psychiatric syndromes'. *Psychiatric Clinics of North America* **12**(1): 89–100.

Hemphill, R. E. (1952) 'Incidence and Nature of Puerperal Psychiatric Illness.' *British Medical Journal* **2**: 1232.

Kempe, M. (1989) (translated by B. A. Windaett, originally published in 1400) *The Book of Margery Kempe* (London: Penguin).

Kendell, R. E., Mackenzie, W. E., West, C., McGuire, R. J. and Cox, J. L. (1984) 'Day to Day Changes after Childbirth: Further Data.' *British Journal of Psychiatry* **145**: 620–5.

Kennedy, H. (1992) *Eve Was Framed: Women and British Justice* (London: Chatto and Windus).

Kitzinger, S. (1992) 'Birth and Violence against Women: Generating Hypotheses from Women's Accounts of Unhappiness after Childbirth.' In Roberts, H. (ed.) *Women's Health Matters* (London: Routledge).

Kramer, H. and Sprenger, J. (orig. 1486) *Malleus Malificarum* (The Hammer of Witches) (reproduced 1948, London: The Pushkin Press).

Liddiard, M. (1923) *The Mothercraft Manual* (London: Churchill).

Lloyd, G. E. R. (ed.) (1978) *Hippocratic Writings* (London: Penguin).

Llewelyn-Davies, M. (1978) *Maternity Letters from Working Women* (London: Virago).

Marcé, L. V. (1858) *Traite de la Folie des Femmes Enceintes, des Nouvelles Accouchées et des Novices* (Paris: Baillière Tindall).

Mead, M. (1971) *Pregnancy, Birth and the Newborn Baby* (New York: Delacote Press, Seymour/Lawrence).

The Motherhood Book: For the Expectant Mother – and Baby's First Years (1949) 'Compiled by a distinguished group of experts' (London: Amalgamated Press).

Napier, R. (1981) (Cited in MacDonald, M., *Mystical Bedlam: Madness Anxiety and Healing in 17th Century England*, (Cambridge: Cambridge University Press).

O'Hara, M. W. and Zekoski, E. M. (1988) 'Postpartum Depression: A Comprehensive Review.' In Kumar, R. and Brockington, I. F. (eds) *Motherhood and Mental Illness*, 2 (London: Wright).

Oakley, A. (1979) *Becoming a Mother* (Oxford: Martin Robertson).

Paykel, E. S. (1980) 'Life Events and Social Support in Puerperal Depression.' *British Journal of Psychiatry* **114**: 1325–35.

Peel Report (1970) *Domiciliary Midwifery and Maternity Bed Needs*. Standing Maternity and Midwifery Advisory Committee Report (London: HMSO).

Platz, C. and Kendell, R.E. (1988) 'A matched-control follow-up and family study of puerpal psychoses.' *British Journal of Psychiatry* **153**: 90–4.

Richardson, D. (1993) *Motherhood and Childrearing* (London: Macmillan).

Rutter, M. (1966) *Maternal Deprivation Re-assessed* (Harmondsworth: Penguin).

Shorter, E. (1991) *Women's Bodies: A Social History of Women's Encounters with Health, Ill Health and Medicine* (London: Transaction).

Showalter, E. (1987) *The Female Malady: Women, Madness and English Culture 1830–1980* (London: Virago).

Solomons, B. (1931) 'Maternal Sepsis and Psychosis.' *Journal of Mental Health* **77**: 707.

Ussher, J. M. (1991) *Women's Madness: Misogyny or Mental Illness* (London: Harvester/Wheatsheaf).

Welburn, V. (1980) *Postnatal Depression* (Manchester: Manchester University Press).

Winterton Report (1992) *Health Committee Second Report on the Maternity Services*, vol. 1. (London: HMSO).

Yalom, I. D., Lunde, D. J., Moor, H. and Hamberg, B. A. (1968) 'Postpartum Blues Syndrome: A Description and Related Variables.' *Archives of General Psychiatry* **18**: 16–27.

Chapter 2

Distressing Events Occurring At or Around the Time of Childbirth

Understanding postpartum emotional disturbance is to remember the mother's unstable hormonal status... to look at her previous psychiatric history... and to see her private childbirth experience as related to certain obstetrical practices and hospital routines.

(Thune-Larsen and Møller-Pedersen, 1988, p. 238)

This chapter is concerned with the relationship between events occurring at or around the time of childbirth and maternal distress and depression. The chapter commences with a consideration of the organic model of postnatal depression developed by Dalton. The major components of this model were summarised in 1984. Organic models of psychiatric disturbance hold that all psychiatric conditions are the result of some underlying physical condition. Consequently, the role of progesterone in postpartum blues and postnatal depression will be considered here. The prophylactic use of progesterone will also be considered in this part of the chapter. However, it will be suggested that Dalton's model fails to take into account the importance of the context in which childbirth takes place.

The second part of the chapter is concerned with the role of the medicalisation and pathologisation of pregnancy and childbirth in the development of postnatal depression and maternal distress. Research concerning the relationship between high levels of medical intervention and postpartum depression and distress will be considered here.

The third part of the chapter will be concerned with research about the development of post-traumatic stress disorder (PTSD) in mothers. The more diffuse notion of birth trauma and new models specifically developed to account for distress following childbirth will also be documented. The chapter will conclude with a discussion of the relative strengths and weaknesses of these types of approach to the issues involved with the onset and treatment of maternal distress believed to be caused by events occurring at or around the time of childbirth.

Katharina Dalton's model of postnatal distress

Dalton (1980, 1984, 1985) has developed an organic model of postnatal distress in which the role of progesterone is of paramount importance. Dalton's thesis is that, in some women, postnatal depression is caused by hormonal changes that occur during pregnancy and after childbirth. Following conception, there is an increase in progesterone. During the second part of a pregnancy, a woman's blood progesterone level may reach between 3 and 50 times the normal level of progesterone found in a healthy menstruating woman on day 21 of her menstrual cycle. In the first part of a pregnancy, this progesterone is produced by the ovaries, but after the 12th week it is produced by the placenta. After the delivery of the baby, the placenta is also delivered, thus abruptly reducing the supply of progesterone. As Hamilton (1989) has indicated, psychiatric symptoms after childbearing tend to arrange themselves into well-defined patterns or syndromes. Many postpartum symptoms and the timing of their development lead to the hypothesis that critical aetiological mechanisms may be related to postpartum hormonal changes. Dalton's work fits within this pattern.

Dalton (1984) is of the opinion that some women are particularly sensitive to hormonal changes and, consequently, find this sudden alteration of hormonal levels difficult to accommodate. It is these women who are at risk of developing postnatal depression. Dalton suggests that the postnatal blues that are experienced by many women may represent a milder, and in most instances transitory, reaction to this sudden change in the level of progesterone.

It is possible, as Dalton (1984) has done, to identify several risk factors that may be indicative of a predisposition to develop postnatal depression. These risk factors are as follows:

- A genetic factor; for example, women whose mother or monozygotic twin has suffered from postnatal depression;
- Age between 20 and 30 years;
- Feeling elated and in excellent health during late pregnancy;

- A pregnancy that has progressed to full term following the possibility of abortion;
- The presence of premenstrual syndrome;
- Postnatal depression in connection with a previous pregnancy.

Although Dalton (1984) points out that stillbirth, neonatal death, obstetric difficulties and epidural deliveries are not risk factors in themselves, it is difficult, given her general theoretical perspective, to understand why this should not be the case in an otherwise 'at-risk' woman. Certainly, the underlying sensitivity to hormonal change would be overlaid by evidence of physical trauma and/or grief, but it is difficult to see why it should not occur in these instances.

Dalton goes on to identify points of onset of maternal distress. These points of onset are as follows:

- Immediately after delivery (all cases of postnatal blues and many cases of postnatal psychosis);
- On stopping lactation;
- On starting hormonal contraception;
- A few days prior to, or with, the first menstruation following childbirth;
- Following the termination of a pregnancy.

Dalton is of the belief that, in most women, the postnatal blues are self-limiting and disappear within the first 2 weeks following delivery. Even in cases in which the symptoms of postnatal depression or postnatal psychosis are present, Dalton (1984) states that, in many women, these symptoms will end with the resumption of menstruation. However, for 'at-risk' women, the symptoms may continue for years.

In *Depression After Childbirth* (1980), Dalton adapts Marcé's (1858) observations and produces an analysis of postnatal depression that links this experience with that of the premenstrual syndrome. Dalton's analysis suggests that, upon recovery from postnatal depression, a woman can go on to experience the premenstrual syndrome, that is, the presence of recurrent symptoms prior to menstruation coupled with the complete absence of symptoms in the postmenstruum. These experiences may continue until the menopause.

Dalton (1980) produces a stage analysis of how postnatal depression may resolve itself into premenstrual syndrome. The three stages she proposes are as shown in Table 2.1. Dalton argues that this type of depression may be distinguished from typical depression owing to the occurrence of marked irritability, weight gain, increased appetite

29

and a persistent yearning for sleep. However, the extent to which these experiences are common to mothers who are not depressed, or are absent from typical depression because the typically depressed do not have a baby to cope with, is open to conjecture.

Table 2.1 Three stages of postnatal depression/premenstrual syndrome

Stage 1 *Postnatal Depression*	The degree of depression is typically severe. This depression may end with the resumption of menstruation; alternatively, it may continue for years.
Stage 2 *Fluctuating Postnatal Depression*	The degree of depression fluctuates. The base line level of depression remains moderate but the degree of depression increases in severity before menstruation and eases back to a more moderate level of depression after menstruation.
Stage 3 *Premenstrual Syndrome*	Any depression is now associated with the premenstrual period. Prior to menstruation the level of depression is severe but there is no depression after menstruation. Premenstrual syndrome may continue until the menopause.

Adapted from Dalton (1980).

Whilst it must be said that Dalton's findings have not always been confirmed by other researchers (for example, Nott *et al.*, 1976), her work would appear to be useful in connection with the prophylactic treatment of women who have already experienced an episode of postnatal depression. As Dalton herself indicates:

> 68% had a subsequent postnatal depression. The recurrence rate was lowest (58%) for those whose first postnatal illness only required treatment by their general practitioner, but it rose to 84% for those who required hospital admission for their first illness.
>
> *(Dalton, 1984, p. 3)*

Clearly, if a subsequent episode of postnatal depression can be avoided, prophylactic measures are indicated. The prophylactic treatment of postnatal depression is aimed at the elimination of a sudden drop in progesterone in the post-delivery period. Its aim is to allow a more gradual return to the levels of progesterone normally found in women who are not pregnant. Consequently, progesterone, in varying doses, is administered for 2 months after the birth or until the return of menstruation, whichever is the earlier.

This method may also be used in the treatment of established postnatal depression. Progesterone can be used in conjunction with psychotropic and antidepressant drugs. Using such a method of treatment, the dosage of psychotropic/antidepressant drugs should, when improvement occurs, be reduced each postmenstruum whilst progesterone therapy is continued from ovulation to menstruation (as in the treatment of premenstrual syndrome). Eventually, the course of progesterone may be gradually reduced, both in length and in dosage, until the woman becomes symptom-free without medication.

Dalton (1985) reports that out of 100 women who requested progesterone prophylaxis during a pregnancy following a previous episode of postnatal depression, only nine experienced a recurrence of postnatal depression. Given the previously reported recurrence rate of 68 per cent in an untreated sample, it would appear that, for the right women, Dalton's treatment may have much to offer.

However, numerous researchers have cast doubt over Dalton's findings. For example, Vandermeer et al. (1984) point out that Dalton's work concerning the prophylatic properties of progesterone was not subjected to a 'double blind' trial. In conducting such a trial themselves, they were unable to replicate Dalton's findings. In particular, they found no difference between the effect of progresterone and the effect of a placebo in their study.

Furthermore, Quadagno et al. (1986) took a sample of 21 couples from childbirth classes and administered questionnaires that assessed 20 different mood states in the third trimester of pregnancy, in the postpartum period and at 6 months post-delivery. Both men and women participated in this study. The results showed that, in many ways, this period was an emotionally unique time and that both the men and the women in their sample tended to experience the postpartum period in an emotionally similar way.

A prospective study conducted by Leverton and Elliott (1989) identified a 'high-risk' group of pregnant women, including those believed to be at risk of developing postnatal depression. Half of their sample were offered preparation for parenthood classes, together with individual support and training in stress management. The other half of their sample acted as a control group. The prevalence of postnatal depression in the group offered the intervention was 19 per cent. Alternatively, the prevalence of postnatal depression amongst the control group was 40 per cent. All of these findings serve to cast doubt upon the overriding influence of hormonal changes in the development of postnatal depression.

Furthermore, equally as many researchers have cast doubt upon the apparently 'normal' occurrence of the allegedly hormonally induced occurrence of postnatal blues. For example, Levy (1987) used a self-rating 'blues' questionnaire that compared women who had experienced childbirth with women who had undergone surgery. Levy found that a period of dysphoria was experienced by both groups.

Also, McIntosh (1986) found that the occurrence of the 'blues' was strongly related to lack of previous experience with babies, implying that additional stress and anxiety might contribute to these occurrences. Certainly, it has long been noted (for example, Yalom *et al.*, 1968; Nott *et al.*, 1976; Priest, 1979) that there is a higher incidence of the blues amongst first-time mothers.

Alternatively, Cone (1972) found that the occurrence of the blues was related to hospital births. Specifically, 64 per cent of those women delivered in hospital experienced 'weepiness', compared with only 19 per cent of women who had their babies at home. Furthermore, other writers (for example, Breen, 1975; Oakley, 1980; Welburn, 1980) have identified specific aspects of hospitalisation, which, they claim, are causally implicated in the development of postpartum blues. These factors include the following:

- Separation from home and family;
- Inflexibility of ward routines;
- Impatient and unsympathetic staff;
- Poor communication;
- Conflict between mother and staff.

One third of the women in Oakley's study and two-thirds of the women in McIntosh's study directly attributed their blues to their experiences during their period of hospitalisation.

McIntosh (1986) proposed that it is highly likely that postnatal blues are multicausal. If this is so, a possible explanation would be that they are the product of stressful features in the postnatal environment acting upon an emotional state already made vulnerable by certain physiological changes occurring in the mother at the time. Specifically, the adoption of this perspective assumes that the action of hormonal or chemical activity is largely that of a predisposing agent. Therefore, distress is not inevitable and may be controlled or reduced by more adequate preparation for infant care and closer attention being paid to the quality of the environment within which labour and postpartum care takes place.

In addition, many authors have argued that certain medical interventions themselves and/or traumatic maternal experiences at or around the time of birth may be enough to trigger a depressive episode. It is to these explanations of postnatal depression and distress that the next section of the chapter will be devoted.

The medicalisation of pregnancy and childbirth revisited

Interest in the impact of discrete medical procedures upon rates of postnatal depression gathered momentum in the 1970s and 80s when the trend towards the increasing medicalisation of pregnancy and the hospitalisation of childbearing women began to be seriously challenged by the various consumer movements associated with pregnancy and childbirth. As Oakley indicates:

> The period from the early 1970s to the late 1980s stands out as the era of consumer movement in maternity care. There is no doubt that professionals providing maternity care have had to assimilate a sustained attacked on their expertise. Beginning as a protest against high induction rates, this quickly generalised itself to become a complaint about the dominance of the medical model of childbirth, in which pregnancy is a pathology requiring institutionalisation and care by high technology means and women merely vessels for foetal transport.
>
> *(Oakley, 1992, p. 9)*

As we have indicated in Chapter 1, the social control of pregnancy and childbirth has a long history, but what had changed significantly was the extent to which the actual process, and indeed the pace, of labour was being increasingly controlled by, usually male, doctors. These doctors were utilising increasingly available technologies and, arguably, undertaking unnecessary interventions that may have been injurious to the mental, as well as the physical, health of the women who were subjected to them.

Indeed, as many authors have pointed out, undertaking one intervention tends to be associated with an increased risk of precipitating another intervention, that is, a cascade of intervention. Figure 2.1 illustrates this process and is adapted from Inch's (1982) consideration of the cascade of interventions that may follow the induction of labour.

Figure 2.1   The cascade of intervention: an induction (Inch, 1982;
taken from Birthrights, Green Print, Rendlesham, by
permission from the publishers)

Prevalence of induction is associated with an increased risk of
prematurity
↓

The presence of a drip and foetal monitoring necessarily confines the
woman to bed and may increase maternal distress
↓

A cascade of intervention. An induction may lead to foetal distress
and foetal distress may lead to a caesarean section being performed
↓

More analgesia may be required to control the pain associated with
an induced labour
↓

An epidural may be administered to control the pain
↓

A higher risk of a forceps delivery is associated with the use of
epidural analgesia
↓

An episiotomy will then be required
↓

The baby may need to be removed to a neonatal unit
↓

The relationship between mother and baby may be affected

Obviously, if it could be proven that any of these interventions were
associated with an increase in postnatal depression amongst their
recipients, this, in itself, might lead to a review of the relevant procedures. Unfortunately, the results of this line of research are typically
mixed. For example, Thurkettle and Knight (1985) found that the
use of obstetric intervention *was* related to postnatal depression.
However, in the following year, O'Hara (1986) found *no* relationship
between obstetric intervention and the onset of postnatal depression.
The range of probable and potential interventions during labour and
childbirth is given in Appendix III.

A similar pattern was repeated when Thune-Larsen and Møller-
Pedersen (1988) suggested that traumatic births are related to subsequent emotional disturbances involving intense pain and anxiety, loss

of control, dissatisfaction with the experience of childbirth and dissatisfaction with the support of the medical and midwifery staff. Alternatively, Green *et al.* (1988) found that the wellbeing of the woman at the end of the puerperium was not related to the number or types of intervention experienced but to the belief that the 'right' thing had happened. In turn, this belief was related to the quality of information received regarding the reasons for the relevant intervention rather than the intervention itself.

To further confuse an already confusing picture, Cartwright and Murray (1993) found that, on the whole, obstetric risk was unrelated to postnatal depression. However, women with a previous history of obstetric trauma were more likely to experience some degree of postnatal depression with the current pregnancy and birth.

However, whilst the evidence is mixed, presumably due to the differing methods, definitions and foci of the relevant research (Kendall-Thackett and Kaufman-Kanter, 1993), responses to it tend not to be. The relevant debates are often both profoundly gendered and heated. For example:

> The natural childbirth group fails to understand that the practices of medicine consists of the recognition and shortcomings of nature – nature is a bad midwife. Childbirth has become safer because of increasingly sophisticated methods of diagnosis and treatment. With the illogiciality of women these are the very procedures they wish to discard... They insist that birth is a natural phenomenon but, equally, so is death.
>
> *(Francis, 1985, p. 69)*

The somewhat obviously offensive associations between women, nature, poor midwifery and illogicality have been shown by Haste (1993) to imply their opposite, that is, an association between men, culture, good midwifery and logicality! However, it has, of course, long been shown that the safety of the mother during childbirth had improved prior to routine hospitalisation and the associated escalation of medical interventions conducted upon women as a matter of routine practice.

Shuttleworth (1990) is one author amongst many who has argued that the debates surrounding the medicalisation of childbirth have a hidden agenda that has far more to do with cultural ideology than with the health, physical or otherwise, of individual women. The hidden patriarchal agenda that Shuttleworth introduces into the debate is as follows:

- The assertion of patriarchal control of women and their reproductive capacities in general;
- The definition, pathologisation and subsequent control of women's 'unruly' bodies in particular;
- The manipulation of the birth process as if it were an entirely technical event;
- An overwhelming interest in pathological processes or with the potential for such processes to occur, coupled with a corresponding lack of appreciation of the 'normal' process of birth.

Lack of clear evidence coupled with an ideological debate may have been two of the factors that led to researchers with an interest in trauma following childbirth to turn to a relatively well-established definition of trauma, that of PTSD.

Post-traumatic stress disorder and birth trauma

The diagnostic criteria for PTSD are well documented (DSM III R, 1987) and are as follows:

1. The person has experienced an event that is outside the range of usual human experience. Such an event would be markedly distressing to almost anyone.
2. The traumatic event is persistently re-experienced in at least *one* of the following ways:
   - Recurrent and intrusive distressing recollections of the event;
   - Acting or feeling as though the traumatic event were reoccurring. This may include flashbacks of the event in question;
   - Intense psychological stress in connection with events that symbolise or resemble the original traumatic event.
3. Persistent avoidance of stimuli associated with the trauma or numbing of general responsiveness (not present before the trauma). This is indicated by at least *three* of the following:
   - Efforts to avoid thoughts or feelings associated with the traumatic event;
   - Efforts to avoid activities or situations that arouse recollections of the trauma;
   - Inability to remember an important aspect of the trauma (psychogenic amnesia);
   - Markedly diminished interest in significant activities;

- Feelings of detachment or estrangement from others;
- Restricted range of affect;
- Sense of a foreshortened future.
4. Persistent symptoms of increased arousal (not present before the trauma) indicated by at least two of the following:
   - Difficulty in falling or staying asleep;
   - Irritability or outbursts of anger;
   - Difficulty in concentrating;
   - Hypervigilance;
   - Exaggerated startle reflex;
   - Physiological reactivity upon exposure to events that resemble aspects of the traumatic event.

Niven (1986) found that whilst 3–4 years after the event most women could recall childbirth accurately, her findings still suggested that a number of women appeared to suffer a mild form of post-traumatic stress associated with childbirth. Tylden (1990) also noted that women who had adverse experiences relating to childbirth had symptoms of PTSD.

Furthermore, Mènage (1993) has indicated that women who rated highly on the DSM III R criteria for the diagnosis of PTSD also experienced feelings of powerlessness, lack of information, a degree of physical pain, a perceived unsympathetic attitude on the part of others and a lack of clearly understood consent for the interventions carried out. Littlewood's (1993, 1996) research would also indicate, particularly in the instance of stillbirth, that many mothers of stillborn babies experience symptoms that firmly fit the diagnostic criteria for PTSD.

However, difficulties arise with attempts to apply the diagnostic criteria associated with PTSD to distress following a difficult experience of childbirth. Firstly, there is the difficulty, given the inconclusive nature of research concerned with interventions believed to be traumatic, of applying criterion 1: 'The person has experienced an event that is outside the range of usual human experience. Such an event would be markedly distressing for almost anyone.' Whilst, catastrophic birth experiences (for example, life threatening to the mother and/or her child, or the death or impairment of the baby) would fit criterion 1, many of the discrete interventions conducted routinely or otherwise would seem to distress some women but not others. Also, there is evidence (for example, Mènage, 1993) suggesting that there may be more issues involved in maternal distress following childbirth than those covered by the diagnostic criteria associated with PTSD.

These difficulties have led some researchers to attempt to develop the concept of 'birth trauma'. 'Birth trauma' refers to a fundamentally negative birth experience that may be either physical or psychological in origin. However, it must be said that birth trauma often results from a combination of both these factors. The concept is a multifaceted one that can include disturbances in body image following interventions performed by health-care professionals that are perceived in terms of physical mutilation on the part of the mother. Trauma may also result from feelings of betrayal by health-care professionals involved with the birth.

Kendall-Thackett and Kaufman-Kanter (1993) argue that it is these factors which may account for some of the marked differences in research outcomes in this area. Specifically, they suggest that results may vary with the distinct focus of the particular piece of research in question. Where there is no perceived connection between birth trauma and postnatal depression, the focus will typically be on purely objective data, for example the number and/or types of medical intervention that have been documented as having occurred. Alternatively, birth trauma is a complex concept which involves some understanding of the meaning of a *particular* intervention for an *individual* mother. In order further to investigate the concept of birth trauma, Kendall-Thackett and Kaufman-Kanter have developed a conceptual framework that is an adaptation of Finkelhor's (1987) Traumagenics Model. Kendall-Thackett and Kaufman-Kanter's conceptual framework is an attempt to describe negative birth experiences in terms of traumatic stress that represents an expansion of the basic model of PTSD. Specifically, Kendall-Thackett and Kaufman-Kanter's model includes interpersonal factors and identifies what they see as the four main aspects of birth trauma: physical damage, stigmatisation, betrayal and powerlessness. This conceptual framework may be summarised as shown in Table 2.2.

The literature concerning physical damage is of interest. Marut and Mercer (1979) make the point that if a woman feels that she has been damaged by her experiences, the symptoms are likely to be traumatising. Wessel (1983) makes a similar point, that is, physical damage in itself might not actually be traumatising, but it is the woman's interpretation of 'damaging' which may be the important factor. Green et al.'s (1988) work is of relevance here. Their findings would indicate that the wellbeing of a woman following childbirth is not related to the number or types of intervention experienced but to the woman's perception of the 'right' thing having happened. In turn, they relate the perception of the 'rightness' of a given course of action to the quality of information received by the

tions of powerlessness and lack of control. Presumably, Finkelhor's (1987) observations would be equally relevant here, but in this instance depression following trauma would result from loss of trust in oneself and one's ability to influence significant events. Certainly, one of the most consistent predictors of positive birth experiences would seem to be a women's feeling of control over the process of labour and childbirth.

For example, Kitzinger (1987) has argued that power is something that labouring women lack, and Cranley et al. (1982), when comparing women's perceptions of vaginal and caesarean section deliveries, found that maternal perceptions of control over the birth process was associated with a positive birth experience. Furthermore, Trowell (1982), in an exploration of the effects of emergency caesarean sections upon the mother–child relationship, also noted that maternal perceptions of control were associated with positive experiences. The following comments were made by a 34-year-old woman concerning her second experience of an emergency caesarean section:

I really feel as though I was given every possible chance to achieve what I wanted. Nobody forced anything on me. I can only look back positively. Even though I ended up with an emergency caesarean section it was absolutely the right decision. I gave birth the only way I know how.

(Trowell, 1982, p. 46)

It is perhaps within this context that Kitzinger's (1992) observations can be fully comprehended. Kitzinger highlighted similarities between the way in which women describe traumatic birth experiences and the way in which rape victims described their assaults. Lack of consent either being sought or given is an obviously significant factor in both instances. Also, a sense of violation of personhood by others, exacerbated by the treatment of the woman as an object, either to be used sexually or used as a 'fetal vessel' against the woman's own wishes and beliefs about herself, is of relevance in both instances. To be physically damaged, made to feel stigma and shame, to lose one's trust in both others and oneself would seem to be the essence of Kendall-Thackett and Kaufman-Kanter's (1993) understanding of birth trauma. In these circumstances, it may not be too surprising to note that the discourses used by women in connection with their experiences of birth trauma are not dissimilar from the discourses used by women to describe their experiences of rape.

However, if perceptions of powerlessness and lack of control are central factors in the experience of birth trauma, it is unsettling to note that Rothman (1982) and Wertz and Wertz (1989), amongst others, suggest that hospitals actively socialise women into powerlessness utilising various methods. Furthermore, the control of pregnancy and reproduction is not without its other battles for control, battles which also leave the woman, to a greater or lesser extent, in a position of relative powerlessness; consider, for example, the longstanding debates concerning the respective roles of largely male doctors versus largely female midwives. Whilst the impact of the consumer movement described by Oakley (1992), coupled with the recommendations of the Winterton Report (1992), may have an impact in terms of giving women more choice in childbirth, the work of McHugh (1994) would indicate that progress in this area may be slow. Furthermore, it is still unfortunately the case that powerful cultural and professional forces may continue to operate against the effective empowerment of women during pregnancy and childbirth. However, if Affonso and Stichler (1978) and Kitzinger (1975) are correct, it might be expected that these forces will also continue to contribute to the prevalence of birth trauma amongst childbearing women.

Ballard et al. (1995) approach the issue of the onset of traumatic disorders following childbirth from a different perspective. These authors express concern because:

> most cases are probably not being recognised. Some patients appeared to be suffering from a prolonged disability that could impair mother/infant relationships. A prompt apology by hospital staff in cases of adverse incidents might avert some of these protracted sequelae.
>
> *(Ballard et al., 1995, p. 528)*

Unfortunately, a prompt apology may be unlikely to be forthcoming. However, if susceptibility to postnatal depression can be associated with maternal distress following birth experiences that are, or are believed to be, traumatic, there still remains the question of how such experiences are overcome in the apparent absence of immediate detection. Horowitz and Kaltreider (1979) maintain that people process traumatic events through a series of stages as they attempt to integrate the event into their own, previously established, cognitive framework. According to Horowitz and Kaltreider, after the initial reaction phase, people fluctuate between denial and intrusive thoughts. It is only with the benefit of time that individuals manage to work 'through' their trauma and eventually find a meaning for the event that is acceptable to themselves.

The work of Smith (1986) also indicates that, in the processing of trauma, the most dominant stages are denial and intrusive thoughts. Smith identifies the characteristics of denial as involving the avoidance of anything connected with the event, numbness and reduced levels of response to people or important activities. To these, Figley (1986) adds rigidly role-adherent or stereotyped behaviours, daze and inattention. Unfortunately, Affonso and Arizmendi (1986) have found that women who have frequent and recurrent thoughts about labour and delivery are, at least in the first instance, less likely to make a successful postpartum adjustment. Furthermore, Padawer *et al.* (1988) have suggested that denial may lead to some women being asymptomatic in the immediate postpartum period and that birth trauma may take weeks, or even months, to emerge.

Stewart (1982) is less than optimistic concerning the issue of the resolution of trauma. Stewart suggests that women who have suffered one episode of childbirth-related post-traumatic stress are generally reluctant to contemplate another pregnancy. Stewart also suggests that sexual, and if applicable marital, relationships also suffer from the impact of this type of trauma. Alternatively, Wilson and Zigelbaum (1986) found that some women got pregnant again very quickly so that they could 'do it right this time'. However, as Mander (1994) has indicated, undertaking another pregnancy following a traumatic experience of childbirth is not necessarily indicative of any resolution of the initial trauma and may paradoxically compound it. Unfortunately, once established, it would seem that birth trauma, however defined, is likely to produce extreme responses one way or another to its onset.

Conclusion

This chapter has looked at events that occur at or around the time of birth which have been associated with the onset of trauma and/or depression in women after childbirth. The chapter commenced with a discussion of Dalton's model of postnatal distress and the association between low levels of progesterone, the postnatal blues and postnatal depression. The role of prophylactic treatment of at-risk groups was also discussed here. It was argued that, whilst Dalton's model may be valuable, factors other than hormonal influences are clearly implicated in the onset of maternal distress.

The chapter went on to consider the role that the medicalisation and associated pathologisation of pregnancy and childbirth may have had in contributing to an increase in the incidence of depression and distress following childbirth. Whilst evidence regarding the impact of individual types of intervention was contradictory, a growing acknowledgement of the relationship between maternal distress and birth experience led some researchers to consider trauma experienced at, or around the time of birth, to be a type of PTSD. However, whilst PTSD is an appropriate diagnostic category for certain kinds of birth trauma, it was concluded that a great deal of trauma short of a diagnosis of PTSD was being excluded by the adoption of this form of categorisation. Consequently, other approaches to birth trauma were considered. These were specifically designed to account for trauma following childbirth and all identified the centrality of the mother's perception of her experience as well as the physical aspects of trauma. At one level, the debates concerning PTSD and birth trauma are reminiscent of the recollections of the anchoress Margery Kempe that were recorded in Chapter 1. Margery, in attempting to account for her own state of mind following childbirth, was unsure whether it was on the one hand 'expecting the worst' (that is, hell and damnation in Margery's case) or on the other poor social support (the stern attitude of her confessor) that was responsible for her condition. Whichever it was, an understanding of 'expecting the worst' and social support offer opportunities for a more sensitive approach to women during or after a traumatic experience. Also, a better understanding of the interpersonal factors contributing to birth trauma may result in preventive actions and/or intervention programmes being undertaken in this area. The importance of prevention and/or interventions designed to limit trauma were underlined by the final section of this chapter, which focused on the difficulties many women faced in coming to terms with a profoundly distressing experience of childbirth.

However, events that occur at or around the time of birth are not the only, or even the major, events associated with the onset of postnatal depression and/or distress. Psychological explanations of postnatal depression focus upon the mother's internal world and upon her assumptions regarding her interactions with her external world (including her baby). It is these types of explanation of maternal depression and distress which are the subject of Chapter 3.

References

Affonso, D. D. and Stichler, J. F. (1978) 'Exploratory Study of Women's Reactions to Having Caesarean Birth.' *Birth and Family Journal* 5: 88–95.

Affonso, D. D. and Arizmendi, T. G. (1986) 'Disturbances in Postpartum Adaptation and Depressive Symptomatology.' *Journal of Psychosomatic Obstetrics and Gynaecology* 5: 88–92.

Ballard, C. G., Stanley, A. K. and Brockington, I. F. (1995) 'Post-Traumatic Stress Disorder (PTSD) After Childbirth.' *British Journal of Psychiatry* 166: 525–8.

Breen, D. (1975) *The Birth of a First Child* (London: Tavistock).

Cartwright, W. and Murray, L. (1993) 'The Role of Obstetric Factors in Post Partum Depression.' *Journal of Reproductive and Infant Psychology* 11(4): 215–20.

Chalmers, B. E. and Chalmers, B. M. (1986) 'Postpartum Depression During the Transition to Parenthood.' *Development and Psychopathology* 4: 29–47.

Cone, B. A. (1972) 'Puerperal Depression.' In Morris, N. (ed.) *Psychosomatic Medicine in Obstetrics and Gynaecology*, 3rd International Congress (London, Basel: Karger).

Cranley, M. S., Hedahl, K. J. and Pegg, S. H. (1982) 'Women's Perceptions of Vaginal and Caesarian Section Deliveries.' *Nursing Research* 32: 10–15.

Dalton, K. (1980) *Depression After Childbirth* (Oxford: Oxford University Press).

Dalton, K. (1984) *A Guide to Prophylactic Progesterone for Postnatal Depression.* Information leaflet given to GPs and women enquirers.

Dalton, K. (1985) 'Progesterone Prophylaxis used Successfully in Postnatal Depression.' *The Practitioner* 229: 507–8.

DSM III R (1987) The Diagnostic and Statistical Manual (DSM) of the American Psychiatric Association (Washington, DC: American Psychiatric Association).

Figley, C. R., (1986) *Trauma and Its Wake*, vol. 2, *Traumatic Stress Theory: Research and Intervention*: New York: Bruner Mozel.

Finkelhor, D. (1987) 'The Trauma of Child Sexual Abuse: Two Models.' *Journal of Interpersonal Violence* 2: 348–66.

Francis, H. (1985) 'Obstetrics: A Consumer Orientated Service? The Case Against.' *Maternal and Child Health* 10: 3–69.

Goffman, I. (1968) *Stigma: Notes on the Management of a Spoiled Identity* (Harmondsworth: Penguin).

Green, J. M., Coupland, V. A. and Kitzinger, J. V. (1988) *Great Expectations: A Prospective Study of Women's Experience of Childbirth* (Cambridge: Childcare and Development Group).

Hamilton, J. A. (1989) 'Postpartum Psychiatric Syndromes.' *Psychiatric Clinicians of North America* 12(1): 89–100.

Haste, H. (1993) *The Sexual Metaphor* (Hemel Hempstead: Harvester/ Wheatsheaf).

Horowitz, M. J. and Kaltreider, N. B. (1979) 'Brief Therapy of Stress Response Syndrome.' *Psychiatric Clinics of North America* **2**: 365–77.

Inch, S. (1982) *Birthrights* (Rendlesham: Green Print).

Janoff-Bulman R. (1986) 'The Aftermath of Victimisation: Rebuilding Shattered Assumptions.' In Figley, C. R. (ed.) *Trauma and its Wake*, vol. 2, *Traumatic Stress Theory: Research and Intervention* (New York: Bruner Mozel).

Kendall-Thackett, K. A. and Kaufman-Kanter, G. (1993) *Postpartum Depression: A Comprehensive Approach for Nurses* (London/Newbury Park, CA: Sage).

Kitzinger, J. (1975) 'The Fourth Trimester.' *Midwife, Health Visitor and Community Nurse* **11**: 118–21.

Kitzinger, S. D. (1987) *Your Baby, Your Way: Making Pregnancy Decisions and Birth Plans* (New York: Pantheon).

Kitzinger, S.D. (1992) 'Birth and Violence Against Women: Generating Hypotheses from Women's Accounts of Unhappiness after Childbirth.' In Roberts, H. (ed.) *Women's Health Matters* (London: Routledge).

Leverton, T. J. and Elliot, S. A. (1989) 'Transition to Parenthood Groups: A Preventative Intervention for Postnatal Depression.' In Hall, E. V. and Everaerd, W. (eds) *The Free Woman: Women's Health in the 1990s* (Carnforth: Parthenon Press).

Levy, V. (1987) 'The Maternity Blues in Post Partum and Postoperative Women.' *British Journal of Psychiatry* **151**: 368–72.

Littlewood, J. (1993) 'The Death of a Premature Baby: Parental Experiences of Bereavement.' Unpublished paper presented to The Society for Reproductive and Infant Psychology's Symposium on Premature Birth, University of Loughborough, 2 April.

Littlewood, J. (1996) 'Stillbirth and Neonatal Death.' In Niven, C. and Walker, A. (eds.) *The Psychology of Reproduction*, vol. 2 (London: Butterworth Heinmann).

Mander, R. (1994) *Loss and Bereavement in Childbearing* (London: Blackwell Scientific).

Marcé, L. V. (1858) *Traite de la Folie des Femmes Enceintes, des Nouvelles Accouchées et des Novices* (Paris: Baillière Tindall).

Marut, J. S. and Mercer, R. T. (1979) 'Comparison of Primiparas' Perceptions of Vaginal and Caesarean Births.' *Nursing Research* **28**: 260–6.

McHugh, N. (1994) 'Bumps a Daisy: Images of Women in AnteNatal Clinic Literature.' Paper delivered to the 24th Annual Conference of the Society for Reproductive and Infant Psychology, September 94, Dublin.

McIntosh, J. (1986) ' Postnatal Blues: A BioSocial Phenomenon?' *Midwifery* **2**: 187–92.

Mènage, J. (1993) 'Post Traumatic Stress Disorder in Women who Have Undergone Obstetric and/or Gynaecological Procedures.' *Journal of Reproductive and Infant Psychology* **11**(4): 221–8.

Niven, C. (1986) 'Labour Pain: Long Term Recall and Consequences.' *Journal of Reproductive and Infant Psychology* **6**: 83–7.

Nott, P. N., Franklin, M., Armitage, C. and Bebler, M. G. (1976) 'Hormonal Changes in Mood in the Puerperium.' *British Journal of Psychiatry* **128**: 379–83.

Oakley, A. (1980) *Women Confined: Towards a Sociology of Childbirth* (Oxford: Martin Robertson).

Oakley, A., 'The Changing Social Context of Pregnancy Care.' In Chamberlain, G. and Zander, L. (eds) *Pregnancy Care in the 1990s* (Parthenon Publishing Group, 1992).

O'Hara, M. W. (1986) 'Social Support, Life Events and Depression During Pregnancy and the Puerperium.' *Archives of General Psychiatry* **43**: 569–73.

Padawer, J. A., Fagen, C., Jannoff-Bulman, R., Steickland, B. R. and Chorowski, M. (1988) 'Women's Psychological Adjustment Following Emergency Caesarian Section versus Vaginal Delivery.' *Psychology of Women Quarterly* **12**: 25–34.

Priest, R. (1979) 'Puerperal Depression and its Treatment.' *The Journal of Maternal and Child Health* August: 312–17.

Quadagno, D. M., Dixon, L. A., Denney, N. W. and Buck, H. W. (1986) 'Postpartum Moods in Men and Women.' *American Journal of Obstetrics and Gynaecology* **154**(5): 1018–22.

Rothman, B. K. (1982) *Giving Birth: Alternatives in Childbirth* (New York: Penguin).

Shuttleworth, S. (1990) 'Women and the Discourses of Sciences.' In Jacobus, M. and Fox-Keller, E. (eds) *Body Politics* (London: Routledge).

Silver, S. M. (1956) 'An Inpatient Programme for Post-Traumatic Stress Disorder.' In Figley, C. R. (ed.) *Trauma and Its Wake*, vol. 2, *Traumatic Stress Theory: Research and Intervention* (New York: Bruner Mozel).

Smith, J. R. (1986) 'Sealing Over and Integration Models of Resolution in the Post Traumatic Stress Recovery Process.' In Figley, C. R. (ed.) *Trauma and Its Wake*, vol. 2, *Traumatic Stress Theory: Research and Intervention* (New York: Bruner Mozel).

Stewart, D. E. (1982) 'Psychiatric Symptoms Following Attempted Natural Childbirth.' *Canadian Medical Association Journal* **127**: 713–16.

Taylor, L. (1992) Maternal Experiences of Premature Birth. Unpublished MA thesis, University of Loughborough.

Thune-Larsen, K. and Møller-Pederson, K. (1988) 'Childbirth Experience and Postpartum Emotional Disturbance.' *Journal of Reproductive and Infant Psychology* **6**: 229–40.

Thurkettle, J. A. and Knight, R. G. (1985) 'The Psychological Precipitants of Transient Post Partum Depression: A Review.' *Current Psychological Research Reviews* **4**: 143–66.

Tilden, V. P. and Lipson, L. G. (1981) 'Caesarean Birth, Variables Affecting Psychological Impact.' *Western Journal of Nursing Research* **3**: 127–49.

Trowell, J. (1982) 'Possible Effects of Emergency Caesarian Section: A Research Study of the Mother/Child Relationship.' *Early Human Development* **7**: 41–51.

Tylden, E. (1990) 'Post-Traumatic Stress Disorder in Obstetrics.' Paper presented at the Fifth International Conference of the Marcé Society of Childbirth and Mental Health, Edinburgh, September.

Vandermeer, Y. G., Loendersloot, E. W. and Van Loenen, A. C. (1984) 'Effect of High Dose Progesterone in Post Partum Depression.' *Journal of Psychosomatic Obstetrics and Gynaecology* **3**: 67–8.

Welburn, V. (1980) *Postnatal Depression* (Manchester: Manchester University Press).

Wertz, R. W. and Wertz, D. C. (1989) *A History of Childbirth in America* (Yale: Yale University Press).

Wessel, H. (1983) *Natural Childbirth and the Christian Family* (New York: Harper Row).

Wilson, J. P. and Zigelbaum, S. D. (1986) 'Post–Traumatic Stress Disorder and the Disposition towards Criminal Behaviour.' In Figley, C. R. (ed.) *Trauma and Its Wake*, vol. 2, *Traumatic Stress Theory: Research and Intervention* (New York: Bruner Mozel).

Yalom, I. D., Lunde, D. J., Moor, H. and Hamberg, B. A. (1968) Postpartum Blues Syndrome: A Description and Related Variables. *Achives of General Psychiatry* **18**: 16–27.

Chapter 3

Psychological Approaches to Distress and Depression Following Childbirth

This Russian-doll imagery of mothers and daughters one inside the other rekindles early anxieties and unresolved issues of love and hate between the pregnant woman and her internal mother (rather than the real one, who may or may not be, alive).

(Raphael-Leff, 1993, p. 80)

This chapter is concerned with the various psychological explanations that have been forwarded as explanations of depression and distress arising during pregnancy and/or following childbirth. The chapter commences with a consideration of psychotherapeutic approaches to depression and distress. These approaches emphasise the importance of early childhood experiences, particularly, in this instance, of a woman's perceptions concerning her relationship with her own mother, to the onset of depression and distress during pregnancy and following childbearing. The many critiques of the psychotherapeutic approach will also be discussed in this part of the chapter.

The second part of the chapter focuses upon attachment theory and mother–infant bonding. Attachment theory emphasises the importance of mother–infant contact, whilst mother–infant bonding is thought to secure the attachment that facilitates a wanted contact between a mother and her baby. It will be suggested here that contemporary evidence would seem to indicate that women who are 'getting to know' their babies use a range of extremely complex strategies that do not seem to be adequately appreciated by some of the proponents of 'bonding' theory. The impact of 'lay' notions of bonding will also be discussed here.

The third part of the chapter is concerned with various cognitive orientations towards the origins of depression and distress. Cognitive orientations emphasise the importance of patterns of thought and differences in indiviudal perceptions. The helpfulness, or otherwise, of congnitive therapy will be discussed here. Finally, a consideration of the problems associated with purely psychological approaches to what is in fact a major life event will conclude the chapter.

Psychotherapeutic approaches to postnatal depression and distress

Psychotherapeutic approaches to maternal distress and depression have a relatively long history and are concerned with the role of the woman's early childhood experiences, particularly her experience of her own mother's mothering. However, many of the findings of those who adopt this perspective have been criticised on the grounds that they pathologise women in general and mothers in particular. Psychcotherapeutic approaches assert the primacy of an individual's experiences and her perceptions of the early stages of her life. Since mothers are frequently central to those experiences, the pathologisation of mothers is a trap into which it is relatively easy to fall. This point is certainly not lost upon Ussher, who indicates that:

> The mother has been a convenient scapegoat throughout the centuries, but psychology and psychiatry have elevated mother hating and mother baiting to the status of scientific fact.
>
> *(Ussher, 1991, p. 184)*

Price (1988) makes a similar point and further suggests that this tendency is especially true of the world of psychoanalysis, where essentially male notions of what constitutes a 'mature' woman (for 'mature' read one that is perceived adequately to service men) abound. Price goes on to argue that, until relatively recently, predominantly male theorists have defined (in the necessary absence of any personal experience of the transition to motherhood) exactly what mothering is, what mothering should hope to achieve and what women should do in order to be judged, presumably by men like themselves, as good mothers. Price is of the opinion that this masculine view of motherhood is essentially primitive in as much as it is usually applied without the advantage of sufficient adult reflection concerning exactly what motherhood is and what mothering entails from the perspective of the mother rather than the child.

Indeed, it would seem to be the case that researchers who have specifically concerned themselves with maternal distress have been somewhat less than woman-centred in their approach. For example, Jannson (1964) looked at the relationship between mental illness and childbirth and put forward the idea that mothers with postnatal depression have a personality defect that relates directly to their sexual and reproductive life. Furthermore, Jannson (1964) argued that postnatal depression was a result of the suppression of latent homosexual tendencies, which were in turn associated with the failure to make a full transition to 'full' womanhood and 'true' femininity. The somewhat dubious beliefs that women can only make a full transition to womanhood via sexuality and maternity are so typical of the patriarchal culture from which they arise that they do not warrant further discussion. The impact of such beliefs upon women will be dealt with fully in Chapter 5.

Nillson and Almgren (1970), in a slightly later study, rated women with postnatal depression on a scale of femininity and concluded that postnatal depression was related to a woman's rejection of her role in childbirth. It is not made clear, however, exactly who defines what that role is. For example, is it the woman's definition, the psychoanalyst's or that of the health-care professionals in attendance at the birth?

As Baker-Miller (1976) has indicated, it is easier to blame individual mothers than to attempt to comprehend an entire system that restricts women on a day-to-day basis as a matter of course. Furthermore, whilst it may be true to say that mothers interact the most with young children and thus may be the most direct agents of systematic cultural oppression, this does not negate the fact that mothers are themselves victims of the system they perpetuate, women who:

> have been deprived and devalued and conscripted as agents of a system that diminished all women.
>
> *(Baker-Miller, 1976, p. 139)*

Irigaray (1980) makes a similar point when she suggests that mothers may simply reproduce the oppression to which they have been subjected. Price (1988) takes these points further and argues that it is only in the eyes of literal or figurative children that mothers *seem* to be all-powerful figures. In fact, most women who are mothers are powerless to change the culture in which they find themselves located.

However, it must be said that not all of those who adopt a psychotherapeutic perspective seek to pathologise, prescribe behaviour or provoke guilt. In an early piece of work, Deutsch (1947) highlighted the importance of a sense of identification that can occur during pregnancy and childbirth between a woman, her mother and her baby. Deutsch was of the belief that where a mother had a hostile relationship with her own mother, she might experience difficulty in identifying with her baby and with acting as a mother. Wolkind *et al.* (1976) continues this theme by putting forward the idea that women deprived of affection and attention in their own childhood experienced difficulties when they became mothers themselves.

However, it is Price (1988) and Raphael-Leff (1991, 1993) who utilise insights derived from psychotherapeutic approaches to delineate the range of the more usual responses to pregnancy and childbirth. Price (1988) considers pregnancy and childbirth to be major psychosocial transitions during which women review their experiences of their own mother and mothering. Such a review often entails a consideration of potentially distressing material that the woman had previously 'filtered out' of her consciousness. Obviously, the more difficult and painful such material is to deal with, the more difficult the individual woman's transition will be. However, Price is optimistic concerning the eventual outcomes of such a review for most mothers. She argues that the process, while potentially distressing, eventually involves the development of a deeper understanding of the actual nature of motherhood as a 'lived in' experience rather than an ideal, or not so ideal, 'type'.

However, this is not to say that the nature of some material reviewed during pregnancy and childbirth may not be profoundly distressing and/or injurious to the woman's subsequent mental health. For example, Rhodes and Hutchinson (1994) describe the labour experiences of survivors of childhood sexual abuse. The women in Rhodes and Hutchinson's study reported both 'forgetting' and 'remembering' the relevant abusive incidents and described their labour sensations as reminiscent of sexual abuse. Rhodes and Hutchinson suggest that styles of labour associated with past experiences of sexual abuse involve the woman fighting, taking control, surrendering and retreating. This style of labouring is considered by Rhodes and Hutchinson to be an extreme of women's reactions to labour in general and to be directly linked to the development of PTSD.

Raphael-Leff (1991, 1993) also considers the review of previous experiences of mothering in her work. Raphael-Leff argues that women carry their experiences of 'mother' within them and may actively respond to any imperfections they perceive in terms of their own interaction with their babies:

each mother differs in the degree to which she has come to terms with the imperfections of early experience and the mother she carries within herself. More emotionally mature women, content to be 'good enough' mothers have found ways of resolving unrealistic idealisation or resentful derogation of their mothers while others still maintain old resentments and skewed expectations about motherhood and are determined to be different or better than their own mothers. Young mothers oscillating between insecurity and over compensatory self confidence may be categorised as over indulgent, over solicitous, over protective and/or perfectionistic.

(Raphael-Leff, 1991, p. 326)

In a later piece of work Raphael-Leff expands upon a system of beliefs that underpin what she refers to as parental orientation. Table 3.1 summarises the parental orientations she identifies.

Table 3.1 Parental orientation and system of beliefs

Belief system	Parental Orientation		
	Facilitator	Reciprocator	Regulator
Adjustment to new baby	Mother adapts	Negotiation	Baby adapts
Basis of adjustment	Baby know best	Inter-subjectivity	Detachment
Beliefs about the baby	Sociable	Different levels of alertness	Asocial – presocial
Role of mothering	Processing	Interaction	Socialisation
Goal of mothering	To secure mature independence	To secure lifelong interdependence	To secure independence
Unconscious attribution	Baby is ideal self	Baby is a person	Baby is repudiated self
Fears/ acceptance	Fear of hating	Acceptance of ambivalence	Fear of loving

Adapted from Raphael-Leff (1991).

Raphael-Leff's work shares similarities with Klein's (1942) observations concerning human development in general. Klein suggested that all babies develop from viewing mother as 'all good' or 'all bad' towards maintaining what she called the 'depressive position', which involves the ability to tolerate the ambivalence inherent in all human relationships. Furthermore, reciprocator mothers share similarities with

Winnicott's (1965) conceptualisation of 'good enough' mothers – mothers who, Winnicott believed, helped the babies' 'true self' (rather than a 'false self' designed to please others) to emerge.

Welldon (1988), in commentating upon an earlier version of Raphael-Leff's observations concerning 'regulator' versus 'facilitator' parental orientations, was concerned, given the nature of her psychotherapeutic practice, with extreme parental orientations. Specifically, she speculates:

It seems to me that in women with severe psychopathology, the Facilitator mother who welcomes the infant's intense dependence on her and the exclusive intimacy of their symbiosis is prone, when severely disturbed to be the mother of transvestite, fetishistic or transsexual boys. On the other hand, the Regulator mother could be more prone, again in extreme cases, to be the mother of battered babies.

(Welldon, 1988, p. 79)

To rephrase Welldon's comments in terms of maternal distress, facilitator mothers are likely to be distressed by signs of their baby's independence and regulator mothers are likely to be distressed by evidence of their infant's continued dependence. However, Raphael-Leff's work is far more broadly based than an analysis of extreme cases and she identifies a range of potentially distressing losses that she associates with the experience of pregnancy and childbirth in general. She points out that, during pregnancy, many women begin to ascribe characteristics to their babies and actively to anticipate how they will mother this baby. This fantasy or imaginary baby is inevitably lost upon the arrival of the real baby and this in itself may be a source of maternal distress as the woman seeks to accommodate a real baby who may differ markedly from her fantasy child. In particular:

precipitating factors of postnatal depression differ according to each woman's maternal orientation

(Raphael-Leff, 1991, p. 141)

and :

Distress may result not only from external imposition but from an internal mismatch. A woman's self esteem may be jeopardised as she feels herself torn between the orientation she has anticipated prenatally, and the materialisation of her capacities as a mother.

(Raphael-Leff, 1991, p. 142)

Furthermore, the three parental orientations described by Raphael-Leff are not fixed personality traits, and an individual woman may orientate herself differently to her subsequent children depending upon her intrapsychic state. In short, Raphael-Leff describes a situation that is fluid and open to change. Given the situation she describes, there are many factors that may be taken to indicate an elevated risk of developing postnatal depression. The factors she identifies are as follows:

1. Conflicted pregnancies, which include the following:
   - Unplanned pregnancies;
   - Untimely pregnancies;
   - 'Wrong' mother, father or baby;
   - Acute ambivalence associated with a pregnancy;
   - Bipolar conflicts associated with extreme 'facilitator' and 'regulator' orientations;
   - Psychosomatic discharge.
2. Emotionally sensitising experiences of the mother, including:
   - Postinfertility pregnancy; [1]
   - A family history of perinatal complications;
   - Borderline personality disorder in the mother;
   - Neurotic defences in the mother;
   - A previous psychiatric history.
3. Complications arising during the pregnancy including:
   - Physical condition of the mother;
   - Other stressful life events associated with the pregnancy;
   - Socioeconomic problems;
   - Lack of emotional support.

Price (1988) adopts a perspective upon parental orientations similar to that of Raphael-Leff and argues strongly that nothing is more harmful to a mother and her baby's emotional futures than early feelings of failure in mothers who are judging themselves and being judged by others in terms of cultural fantasies rather than as ordinary 'good enough' mothers. Price indicates that, for many mothers, anything short of perfection begins to feel like a terrible failure. According to Price, these mothers rapidly become caught up in a downward spiral of trying ever harder to achieve the unachievable and then feel increasingly guilty over what they see as the worst and most unforgivable failure of their whole lives.

From Price's perspective, depression can result from anger being turned against the self rather than aimed at the person who has caused it. She notes that the negative sides of motherhood rarely receive a cultural airing and, consequently, many women are left unprepared for experiences of anger and anxiety following the birth of their baby. Price is of the opinion that anger is a disquieting emotion but that anxiety is one of the most powerfully emotionally wearing experiences of all.

Psychotherapeutic explanations of postnatal depression and maternal distress are relatively common in the relevant literature. As Gilbert (1992) points out, they add much to our understanding of neuroses, but there is unfortunately little evidence to suggest that psychotherapy itself is an effective form of treatment during pregnancy or immediately after childbirth. Nevertheless, the adoption of this perspective would indicate that pregnancy and childbirth are transitions that have a major impact upon the intrapsychic world of the mother. Furthermore, if the woman's intrapsychic world has been damaged in the past in any way, the transition to motherhood may not be a smooth one, irrespective of issues such as duration of labour or type of delivery.

Attachment theory and mother–infant bonding

Whilst psychotherapeutic perspectives are primarily concerned with intrapsychic conflicts that have their origins in childhood, the work of John Bowlby is rather more concerned with the developments of attachment between mothers and babies. In a series of work that commenced in the 1950s he developed an understanding of the origins of attachment and the impact of separation from and/or loss of others to whom one is attached. Bowlby's work has been highly influential in terms of social and hospital policy and is now commonly referred to in the lay literature.

Attachment theory incorporates an evolutionary perspective along with a psychodynamic perspective. The theory rests upon an appreciation of instinctive attachment and response mechanisms. It also rests upon the hypothesis that a child's attachment to his or her mother is mediated by a number of instinctive response systems. Bowlby believed that all relationships of physical and emotional significance are built around the same general pattern, that is, the one that was first developed between mother and baby. To put the theory very simply, a mother's absence provokes certain instinctive responses such as anxiety, protest and searching, whilst a mother's presence terminates them. Bowlby believed that this behaviour was part of our evolutionary heritage as social animals for whom separation from the group could result in physical danger. Furthermore, humans attach themselves to one person (monotropic bonding) rather than to the group as a whole. In these circumstances, it is the loss of one particular person rather than the group as a whole which is the source of distress. Consequently, the presence in the immediate environment of the mother is believed to be of vital importance to the development of her child. Furthermore, at least as the theory was initially expounded, since human infants only bond with one person (that is, their mother), a substitute adult simply will not do. From this perspective, any disruption of the early relationship between mother and child, particularly disruption involving separation, is seen to be a potential source of developmental difficulty for the child and to result in lifelong disruption of an individual's ability to make and break affectional bonds.

Whilst Bowlby's work has been the subject of detailed criticism (for example, Rutter, 1966) and extensive revision, taken within its context the work might be said to have championed the cause of the child. Bowlby's initial observations were made in the period immediately following the wartime separations of many children from their parents across Europe. However, Bowlby's work has also had a less than positive effect upon women. The notions of instinct and bonding have proven particularly problematic when translated via the lay literature to the popular culture. Whilst ideas about maternal instincts certainly did not originate from Bowlby's work, his work did give some further credence to the notion that mothering comes 'naturally' to women. Furthermore, the term 'instinct' can be taken to imply that a woman can mother without any recourse to cognition (always assuming that she has been appropriately mothered herself). Consequently, experience, learning and reflection are all devalued by a biological discourse that asserts the primacy of 'instinctive' behaviour. Furthermore, mothering is portrayed as easy, a preprogrammed rather than an acquired skill. Pity the self-esteem of the woman who finds her 'instincts' let her down!

A similar overly deterministic view emerged concerning the starting point of attachment behaviour, that is, mother–infant bonding. Klaus and Kennell (1976) initially thought that 'bonding' had a 'critical period' (a time when it was particularly easy) of between 6 and 12 hours after birth. They further argued that skin-to-skin contact between mother and baby was extremely important in terms of facilitating the process of mother–infant bonding. Klaus and Kennell found differences in infant behaviour lasting for 2 years when they compared the development of infants who had 'routine hospital access' to their mothers with the development of infants who had routine and extra access to their mothers. Whilst the work of Klaus and Kennell was effective in changing hospital access policies for women and their babies, the work also raised, via its emergence in the 'lay' literature, maternal anxieties over the long-term consequences for their infants of a 'failure' to bond.

Robson and Kumar (1980) indicate that such feelings are quite common but usually last only for a few days. Alternatively, Niven (1992) has argued that a cultural myth of bonding is already in place and that many women expect to experience 'bonding' as part of the 'normal' reaction following childbirth. Niven is of the opinion that a woman's contact with her baby should be determined by the mother's needs and feelings rather than by notions regarding the necessity of 'bonding' within a given period of time.

Alternatively, Brady-Fryer (1994) has noted that multiparas of preterm infants showed both an understanding of bonding and distinct variations in their beliefs about it:

> The terms *bonding* and *attachment* have been used in the professional and lay literature since the 1960's. Study mothers were familiar with the lay interpretation of the concept and compared their developing relationships with their pre-term infants to those established with their previous children.
>
> *(Brady-Fryer, 1994, p. 205)*

Some mothers in Brady-Fryer's study feared bonding with the preterm infant (in case the baby died), others felt that they bonded easily with their infants and still others were uncertain whether or not their babies had bonded with them. Brady-Fryer's study would seem to indicate that a woman's early relationship with her baby is a multifaceted one, one which is dependent upon a number of cues and is not dependent upon skin-to-skin contact occurring at a particular time. Sluckin *et al.* (1983) are particularly scathing about bonding periods:

> no mother should be forced through a ritual bonding period if she is not initially interested in her baby. It may seem far fetched but one can well imagine a situation in which mother and baby bonding becomes a timetabled hospital procedure – the clinical reductio ad absurdum of a compelling but unproven theory.
>
> *(Sluckin et al., 1983, p. 53)*

Eyer (1992) goes further and cites 'bonding' as an example of 'scientific fictionalising'. Whilst Eyer does not imply that bonding researchers fabricated their data, it is argued that these studies were limited by both inadequate research traditions and ideological assumptions about women:

> Perhaps the most profound influence of all on the construction and acceptance of bonding was a deeply embedded ideology regarding the proper role of women.
>
> *(Eyer, 1992, p. 9)*

Overall, attachment theory has indicated the importance of the quality of relationships that babies have with their caregivers and has been successful in changing hospital practices that previously restricted access between women and their children. However, lay notions of 'maternal instincts' and 'bonding' may be counterproductive in as much as an expectation of instinctive homogeneity may overlay patterns of individual variation. The importance of individual variation is one of the central tenets of cognitive approaches to psychology in general and to maternal distress and depression in particular.

Cognitive orientations to depression and distress

Cognitive orientations to depression and distress all focus, to a greater or lesser extent, upon the importance of understanding the meanings and interpretations that different people put on the same events. An early example of such a theory is Kelly's (1955) development of personal construct theory. Kelly was of the opinion that a person's 'self' or personality may be seen in terms of a system of interrelated constructs that inform the individual's attempts to make sense of the external world. Specifically, Kelly asserts that a person looks at the world:

> through transparent patterns or templates which he creates and then attempts to fit over the realities of which the world is composed... Let us give the name constructs to these patterns which are tried on for size. They are ways of construing the world.
>
> *(Kelly, 1995, pp. 8–9)*

According to the theory, constructs are interrelated systems and the sum total of a person's construct system is that person's self. The fundamental postulate of the theory is that 'a person's processes are psychologically channelised by the ways in which they anticipate events'. From this perspective, people react to the past in order to reach out to the future and are actively engaged in a process of perpetual validation that involves checking to see just how much sense their 'self' has made out of the world in terms of how well they can anticipate future events. In short, Kelly's theory indicates the importance of people attempting to impose subjective meaning on the world. Consequently, people develop their own view of the world (that is, a theory concerning what they think it is and how they think it works), their own expectations concerning what is likely to happen in certain situations (hypotheses based upon subjective probabilities) and constantly experiment through their behaviour with life.

Kelly's theory has an associated technique (repertory grid technique) that may be used to delineate aspects of any person's internal world. For example, repertory grid technique could be used to identify and monitor changes in a woman's internal representations of her mother, herself and her actual or fantasy baby. Obviously, such a technique could be of assistance in anticipating any problems that may arise.

In the context of losses associated with the human immunodeficiency virus (HIV), Sherr (1989) and George (1992) criticise the existing accounts of reactions to situations of loss as being overly prescriptive timetables that provide no insight into the unfolding patterns of individual loss and no help in planning care. George's recommendation for more effective counselling combines a systems approach (Jenkins, 1989) with personal construct theory (Bannister and Fransella, 1986). This type of approach offers some structured insight into the meaning that a particular event has for a specific person.

However, whilst personal construct theory focuses upon meaning at an individual level, Beck et al. (1961) have focused upon meanings associated with, in particular, depression. Consequently, Beck et al.'s approach to cognitive therapy deals specifically with cognitions associated with depression. From this perspective, faulty thoughts lead directly to biases in perception, which in turn lead into depression. Beck argued that negative thoughts, based upon previous experience, exist in the form of schemata that are activated when similar events are experienced, thus influencing the interpretation of current events.

These cognitive 'errors' and 'automatic' negative thoughts lead to negative evaluations of self, the world and others and eventually lead to depression. Cognitive 'errors' include the following:

- Arbitrary influences;
- Selective abstraction;
- Overgeneralisation;
- Magnification;
- Minimalisation;

- Personalisation;
- Dichotomous thinking.

Cognitive therapy aims to change these 'automatic' negative thoughts and so help to lift depression.

However, Beck's theory is not without its critics. For example, Lewinsohn *et al.* (1982) question whether negative cognitions are antecedents or simply the consequences of the depression. Smail (1991) questions the laboratory-based experimental approach of cognitive therapy and suggests that all that is revealed are reactions to often bizarre experimental conditions rather than 'everyday' processes of thought. Nevertheless, the focus upon the ways in which different individuals interpret the same event is a valuable one, given the nature of postnatal depression and distress.

Rutter (1966) introduced the concept of 'locus of control' into the relevant literature. The concept of locus of control represents another attempt to define why different people may interpret the same event in different ways. Wallston and Wallston (1981) indicate that an individual's locus of control is an enduring personality quality that transcends the immediate situation and includes the expectation that a person with certain personality characteristics will act in a certain way.

Locus of control comprises a person's perception, developed over many experiences, of what causes things to happen in their lives. The locus of control may be external, when the person tends to blame others or the environment when things go wrong, or it may be internal, when a person blames herself or assumes responsibility for events that may befall her. Dimitrovsky *et al.* (1987) define locus of control in the following way:

- Internal locus of control – a person perceives life events as resulting from his own behaviour;
- External locus of control – events relate to factors beyond personal control, for example chance or the influence of others.

Dimitrovsky *et al.* (1987) found that women with an external locus of control tended to be more emotionally changeable than women with an internal locus of control. They suggest that the vulnerability they found in this group of women pre- and postpartum may lie less in a predisposition to depression than in a tendency to be affected in a more extreme way by the events to which they are exposed.

Seligman (1976) has argued that human depression may be explained in terms of what he called 'learned helplessness'. Learned helplessness is the result of an original state of trauma-induced anxiety being replaced by depression if the person or animal believes that she can neither control nor avoid the trauma. In such a situation, coping behaviours become inhibited and the person or animal enters a phase of withdrawal and inaction.

Abramson *et al.* (1978) modified Seligman's original laboratory-based findings, which involved the administration of actual trauma, to include belief about the control of events. In 1980 Peterson and Seligman identified a particular type of attribution of control over events that they associated with depression in women. According to Peterson and Seligman, when women are depressed bad events are attributed to causes that are believed to be internal, stable and global, whilst good events are attributed to causes that are external, unstable and specific. In an edited collection Gross (1990) cited a particular type of attribution of control over events that was associated with depression in women.

At one level, according to Gross, the findings might be said to cast doubt upon the relevance of the concept of locus of control to a female population already suffering from depression. Specifically, it would appear that the women who were the subjects of the study adopted an external locus of control when things went well and an internal one when things went badly. Furthermore, it might also be argued that women in general may be more likely (a) to experience learned helplessness and (b) to adopt an external locus of control. As Simmons (1987) has noted, young women are more vulnerable to experiences of depersonalisation and loss of self-esteem because of their reliance upon the opinions of others for self-definition. Simmons suggests that this can progress into adulthood if the woman is not given encouragement and valued for what she is rather than the use she can be put to in the service of others. Also, women are less likely than men to adopt active styles of coping with events (Verbrugge, 1985). Indeed, as Haste (1993) has indicated, the cultural association between femininity and passivity is an exceptionally strong one: a woman should not be seen to be able to do anything about anything. Consequently, it might be suggested that relatively large numbers of women adopt an external locus of control and are subsequently more vulnerable to depression as a result. It may be the case that, once a depression has established itself, a woman feels so 'bad' that she begins to attribute bad things happening to her as 'just desserts' and good things happening to her as chance. The difficulty is the same one as Lewinsohn *et al.* (1982) identified in connection with cognitive therapy, that is, it is difficult to know whether the style of attribution is a cause or an effect of the depression.

Another area of research that indicates the importance of a sense of control is life events research. In an early piece of work, Holmes and Rahe (1967) introduced the Social Readjustment Rating Scale. The basic assumption underlying the scale is that stress is created by all events that require change, irrespective of whether the actual event is deemed desirable or undesirable. The Social Readjustment Rating Scale allows the amount of life stress a person has experienced in a given amount of time (for example, 6–12 months) to be measured numerically. Some items from The Social Readjustment Rating Scale are given in Table 3.2. Whilst all change is considered stressful from this perspective, it has been suggested that it is changes that are perceived to be uncontrollable which are associated with the development of depression. Brown (1986) also pointed out that it is the perceived uncontrollability of change which makes it so stressful.

Gross (1990) reports upon an adaption of Rotter's (1966) locus of control scale which included a life events scale. They found that life events stress was more closely related to psychiatric symptoms (especially depression and anxiety) where people rated highly on an external locus of control when compared with those who rated highly on an internal locus of control. It would seem that, if our previous points are accepted, women might be expected to be particularly at risk of developing anxiety or depression in response to life events stress.

Table 3.2 Examples from the Social Readjustment Rating Scale

Rank	Life Event	Mean value
1	Death of Spouse	100
12	Pregnancy	40
13	Sex difficulties	39
14	Gain of new family member	39
16	Change in financial state	38
26	Partner begins or stops work	26
28	Change in living conditions	25
29	Revision of personal habits	24
34	Change in recreation	19
36	Change in social activities	18
38	Change in sleeping habits	16

Data from Holmes and Rahe (1967).

However, whilst pregnancy is clearly a life event stress in itself, it is rapidly followed by others. For example, using the Social Readjustment Rating Scale given in Table 3.2, pregnancy is given a mean value of 40. However, the pregnancy may have resulted in personal illness or injury (53), caused sex difficulties (39), resulted, more often than not, in the gain of a new family member (39) and caused a change in financial state (38). Immediately following these changes, a change to a different line of work may be experienced (36), a 'wife' may restart or stop work (26), personal habits may have to be revised (24), a change in work hours or conditions may be experienced (20), and changes in recreational (19) and social activities (18) may be associated with an almost certain change in sleeping habits (16). It would be difficult to conclude that pregnancy and childbirth do not represent a major life stress for women. Furthermore, the stress would appear to be present and require adjustments for a long period of time. It is hard to disagree with one of Llewelyn-Davies' (1978) respondents quoted in Chapter 1 when she points out that 'the best of times are bad enough'. The psychosocial outcome of the 'best of times' for mothers is recorded in Chapter 4. It is Chapters 7 and 8 that will consider the worst of times.

Conclusion

This chapter has been concerned with psychological approaches to depression following childbirth. It commenced with a consideration of psychotherapeutic approaches to the subject. These approaches focus upon pregnancy as a transition that provokes both a reappraisal of our understanding of mothering together with the possibility of the re-emergence of previously repressed painful experiences. From this perspective, any problems associated with the woman's past, particularly those associated with her own mother's mothering, may be associated with maternal distress and/or depression in the present. An individual woman's orientation towards mothering was identified, and the relationship between different maternal orientations and different distress-provoking events was discussed.

The second part of the chapter looked at attachment theory and mother–infant bonding. From the perspective of attachment theory, separation of the woman from her own mother may be taken to be indicative of a problem. However, it was also indicated that the lay understanding of both attachment and bonding could be sources of maternal distress in themselves.

The third part of the chapter considered the various cognitive explanations of maternal depression and distress. Cognitive styles involving the perception of an inability to control significant life events were identified as problematic from this perspective. However, it was also suggested that pregnancy and childbirth were major life events in themselves, and major life events are associated with distress in themselves irrespective of any notions concerning control. It is the social consequences of adjusting to such a major life event and its relationship to maternal distress and depression that will be the subject of Chapter 4.

Note

1. Whilst most of Raphael-Leff's elevated risk factors for postnatal depression are self-explanatory, postinfertility pregnancies are believed to be potentially problematic because the baby is likely to be perceived as 'extra' precious. Consequently, the pregnancy tends to be overvalued and overmonitored. Also, fear of loss may be strongly felt in postinfertility pregnancies and unfortunately the diagnosis and treatment of infertility can itself result in an erosion of self-esteem.

References

Abramson, L. Y., Seligman, M. E. P. and Teasdale, J. D. (1978) 'Learned Helplessness in Humans: Critique and Reformulation.' *Journal of Abnormal Psychology* **87**: 49–74.

Baker-Miller, J. (1976) *Towards a New Psychology of Women* (London: Pelican).

Bannister, D. and Fransella, F. (1986) *Inquiring Man: The Psychology of Personal Constructs*, 3rd edn (London: Croom Helm).

Beck, A. T. Ward, C. H., Mendelson, M., Mock, J. and Erbaugh, J. (1961) 'An Inventory for Measuring Depression.' *Archives of General Psychiatry* **4**: 561–9.

Brady-Fryer, B. (1994) Becoming the Mother of a Preterm Baby. In Field, P. A. and Marck, P. B. (eds) (1983) *Uncertain Motherhood: Negotiating the Risks of the Childbearing Years* (London: Sage).

Brown, R. (1986) *Social Psychology* (New York: Free Press)

Deutsch, H. (1947) *The Psychology of Women* (New York: Grune and Stratton).

Dimitrovsky, L., Perez-Hirshberg, M. A. and Itskowitz, R. (1987) 'Locus of Control and Depression Pre and Post Partum.' *Journal of Reproductive and Infant Psychology* **5**: 235–44.

Eyer, D. E. (1992) *Mother/Infant Bonding: A Scientific Fiction* (Newhaven and London: University Yale Press).

George, R. J. D. (1992) 'Coping with Death Anxiety – Trying to Make Sense of it All.' *AIDS* **6**: 1037–8.

Gilbert, P. (1992) *Depression: the Evolution of Powerlessness* (Hove: Lawrence Erlbaum).

Gross, R. D. (ed.) (1990) *Psychology: Science of Mind and Behaviour* (London: Hodder and Stoughton).

Haste, H. (1993) *The Sexual Metaphor* (Hemel Hempstead: Harvester/ Wheatsheaf).

Holmes, T. H. and Rahe, R. H. (1967) 'The Social Readjustment Rating Scale.' *Journal of Psychosomatic Research* **II**: 213–18.

Irigaray, L. (1980) 'When our Lips Speak Together.' *Signs* **6**(1): 66–79.

Jannson, B. (1964) 'Psychic Insufficiencies Associated with Childbearing.' *Acta Psychiatrica Scandanavia Suppl.* **220**(9): 141.

Jenkins, E. (1989) 'Handling Loss: A Systems Framework.' *Palliative Medicine* **3**: 97–104.

Kelly, G. A. (1955) *The Psychology of Personal Constructs*, vols 1 and 2 (New York: Norton).

Klaus, M. H. and Kennell, J. H. (1976) *Maternal–Infant Bonding* (St Louis: C. V. Mosby).

Klein, M. (1942) *The Psycho-Analysis of Children* (London: Hogarth/ Institute of Psycho-Analysis).

Lewinsohn, P. M., Steinmetz, J. L. and Larsen, D. W. (1982) 'Depression-Related Cognitions: Antecedent or Consequences.' *Journal of Abnormal Psychology* **90**: 213–19.

Llewelyn-Davies, M. (1978) *Maternity: Letters from Working Women* (London: Virago).

Nillson, A. and Almgren, P. E. (1970) 'Paranatal Emotional Adjustment: A Prospective Study of 165 Women.' *Acta Psychiatrica Scandinavia Suppl.* **220**: 9–41.

Niven, C. A. (1992) *Psychological Care for Families Before, During and After Birth* (London: Butterworth/Heinemann).

Price, J. (1988) *Motherhood: What it Does to your Mind* (London: Pandora).

Raphael-Leff, J. (1991) *Psychological Processes of Childbearing* (London: Chapman & Hall).

Raphael-Leff, J. (1993) *Pregnancy: The Inside Story* (London: Sheldon Press).

Rhodes, N. and Hutchinson, S. (1994) 'Labour Experiences of Childhood Sexual Abuse Survivors.' *Birth* **21**: 213–19.

Robson, K. and Kumar, R. (1980) 'Delayed Onset of Maternal Affection After Childbirth.' *British Journal of Psychiatry* **136**: 347–53.

Rotter, M. (1966) 'Generalised Expectancies for Internal versus External Control of Reinforcement.' *Psychology Monographs* **30**(1): 1–26.

Rutter, M. (1966) *Maternal Deprivation Re-Assessed* (Harmondsworth: Penguin).

Seligman, M. E. P. (1976) *Helplessness: On Depression Development and Death* (San Francisco: W. H. Freeman).

Sherr, L. (ed.) (1989) *Death, Dying and Bereavement* (Oxford: Blackwell Scientific).

Simmons, R. (1987) 'Self-Esteem in Adolescence.' In Holness T. and Yardley K. (eds) *Self and Identity: Perspectives Across the Life Span* (London: Routledge and Kegan Paul).

Sluckin, W., Herbert, M., and Sluckin, A. (1983) *Maternal Bonding* (Oxford, Blackwell).

Smail, D. (1991) 'Towards a Radical Environmentalist Psychology of Help.' *Psychologist* **2**: 61–5.

Ussher, J. M. (1991) *Women's Madness: Misogyny or Mental Illness* (London: Harvester/Wheatsheaf).

Verbrugge, L. (1985) 'Gender and Health: An Update on Hypotheses and Evidence.' *Journal of Health and Social Behaviour* **26**: 156–82).

Wallston, K. A. and Wallston, B. S. (1981) 'Health Locus of Control Scales.' In Lefcourt, H. M. (ed.) *Research with the Locus of Control Construct* (New York: Academic Press).

Welldon, E.V. (1988) *Mother, Madonna, Whore: The Idealisation and Denigration of Motherhood* (London: Guildford Press).

Winnicott, D. W. (1965) *The Family and Individual Development* (London: Tavistock).

Wolkind S. N., Kruk, S. and Chaves, L. P. (1976) 'Childhood Separation Experiences and Psychological States in Primiparous Women: Preliminary Findings.' *British Journal of Psychiatry* **128**: 391–6.

Chapter 4

Sociological Explanations of the Origins of Postnatal Distress and Depression

Rather, what appears to happen is that women experience increased distress and less satisfaction in their relationships particularly with their spouse... taken together with the blues that women frequently experience during the first week postpartum it is clear that women should be prepared for these disturbing changes.

(O'Hara et al., 1990, p. 14)

This chapter is concerned with the social context of maternal distress and depression. The first part of the chapter looks at distress and depression during the early postpartum period. It has been suggested (in Chapter 3) that both pregnancy and childbirth are highly stressful life events, and it would appear that some degree of maternal distress is almost universally present amongst women who have recently given birth. Consequently, the first part of the chapter documents some of the relevant research in this area.

The second part of the chapter is concerned with distress and depression arising from additional burdens of care falling upon the mother. Social and/or environmental factors associated with additional maternal distress will be discussed here. This part of the chapter also includes difficulties of care arising from a more stressful postpartum home environment.

The third part of the chapter is concerned with the association between the experience of motherhood and loss. Whilst the losses associated with loss of identity and self-esteem will be covered here, the issue of role loss will not be fully addressed.

The fourth part of the chapter focuses upon the distinctions drawn by contemporary feminist researchers between depression and oppression. These authors, drawing upon the insights of earlier labelling theorists, strongly argue that postnatal depression is simply a label that is used in order to mask the widespread oppression of women who become mothers in the contemporary social context.

Maternal distress in the early postpartum period

As O'Hara *et al.* (1990) have indicated, life events research should be treated with caution. Specifically, one of the major difficulties in conducting research into major life events is that, in almost all instances, the life event being studied has already occurred, that is, the majority of studies in the area are, by necessity, retrospective. However, childbirth is one of the few major life events that can be predicted with relative certainty and studied prospectively. Consequently, life event research concerned with pregnancy and childbirth is probably more reliable than most research conducted in the general area of the relationship between major life events and the onset of depression and distress.

However, depression is only one indicator of psychological distress and, in the case of pregnancy and childbirth, may be a particularly insensitive one. For example, for a woman to be categorised as suffering from depression, she must display significant mood disturbance and associated symptoms lasting for at least one week. Furthermore, there must be evidence of substantial impairment in role functioning (Spitzer *et al.*, 1978).

Although it is entirely appropriate to adopt restrictive criteria in order clearly to define a major psychological disorder, such criteria may be quite insensitive to an extremely wide range of other forms of psychological distress. However, there have been relatively few studies that focus upon changes in the level of psychological distress and social adjustment through pregnancy and the puerperium (O'Hara and Zekoski, 1988). Furthermore, of the studies that have been conducted, several have found, at least with respect to depressive symptomatology, that women may report less distress, rather than more, after delivery when compared with during pregnancy (see, for example, O'Hara *et al.*, 1982; Elliot *et al.*, 1983). However, without the benefit of a comparison between pregnant women and non-childbearing women, it is extremely difficult to interpret the significance of any of these findings.

One of the few studies that have the benefit of a prospective design and a control group was conducted by O'Hara *et al.* These writers were of the opinion that:

The results of this study leave little doubt that there is some deterioration in women's psychological and social adjustment associated with the latter part of pregnancy and the early puerperium. This deterioration which is largely but not completely remedied by nine weeks postpartum evidently does not result in a significant rise in depression rates.

(O'Hara et al., 1990, p. 14)

O'Hara *et al.* concluded that many women experienced distress and unpleasant changes in their lives in the later stages of pregnancy and the early stages of childrearing. However, they also found that this distress rarely resulted in the woman affected by it seeking any advice or help from professional sources. O'Hara *et al.* suggested that, since distress would appear to be widespread, women should be actively prepared for disturbing and negative changes following the birth of a child in order that they be put into a position to mitigate their effects.

Price (1988) makes a similar, but more expansive, point when she observes that very little attention at all is paid to the 'darker' side of mothering. Consequently, many women are profoundly disturbed by the emotional experiences, particularly those associated with anger and anxiety, which they presumably simply endure.

Alternatively, the positive side of mothering is relatively well documented and widely known. As Doyal indicates:

Mothering at first sight appears to be highly valued work and many find their relationship with their children the most rewarding ones of their lives. Watching them grow can be exhilarating and the unconditional love of young children is immensely pleasurable.

(Doyal, 1995, pp. 38–39)

However, many other authors have identified difficulties and sources of emotional distress. For example, childcare has been shown to be both physically and emotionally demanding (Oakley, 1981; Boulton, 1983; Stevens and Meleis, 1991). For first-time mothers in particular, the responsibility of a new baby can often provoke extreme anxiety, and sleepless nights do little to help the situation. Extreme fatigue is one of the most commonly reported sources of maternal distress.

Also, research has shown that many women suffer from significant physical problems themselves in the aftermath of childbirth (see, for example, Cartwright, 1988; Romito, 1990; Romito and Zaleteo, 1992). In these circumstances, it should not surprise us too much to note that some women become depressed for varying periods (Romito, 1990; Stein *et al.*, 1989).

Doyal (1995) has noted that whilst precise figures are difficult to obtain, it may be the case that postnatal depressions that last for a longer period of time are related to the social and economic circumstances in which the woman mothers. Doyal further suggests that ordinary mothering may be problematic in itself and there may be a continuum between the experiences of mothers who are clinically depressed and those who are not (Romito, 1993).

Additional burdens of care

In their consideration of maternal depression and fatigue Thorpe *et al.* (1991) report that, whilst they found numerous factors to be associated with maternal depression and distress, these findings are, nevertheless, readily interpretable. They suggest that all of their individual findings could be related to indicators of inadequate levels of social support and/or a more stressful postpartum environment. As an example, obvious additional burdens of care fall to women who live alone or to women who become the mothers of twins. Macarthur (1991) suggests that some indirect support for these observations comes from the lower rate of depression found amongst Asian women respondents. Macarthur associates this lower rate of depression with the community support and extended family groups more typically found in this ethnic subculture.

In a much quoted piece of work, Brown and Harris (1976) looked at clinical depression in terms of rates of disorder in particular populations. They sought to explain differences between populations by reference to the everyday lives of the individuals involved. Specifically, they were attempting to link rates of clinical depression to different social class groups and similar broad social categories (including mothers). They began by developing a causal model of depression based on the day-to-day experiences of each woman affected by it.

In this way, Brown and Harris found a large and apparently causal link between life events and depression. They found that many life events were associated with a loss of a sense of life's reality or meaning. Consequently, they associated depression with real or threatened losses. However, they found no evidence that childbirth and pregnancy were specifically related to depression, although it must be said that many of their respondents, particularly working-class women, were prone to depression for other reasons.

Pregnancy and childbirth associated with a severe ongoing problem did increase the risk of clinical depression. Specifically, among the relevant respondents:

- 5 were inadequately housed;
- 5 were experiencing severe marital discord;
- 1 woman was single and opted to have her pregnancy terminated;
- 1 woman suffered a later miscarriage.

Brown and Harris concluded that the experience of pregnancy and childbirth brought home feelings of hopelessness in women by making them particularly aware of the unsatisfactory nature of their position. However, it could also be argued that pregnancy and childbirth are factors that severely limit any chance the woman had, or may have thought she had, of getting out of the position in which she found herself.

Brown and Harris also found that having the care of children was associated with clinical depression. Specifically, working-class women with children at home had a four times greater chance of developing depression when compared with middle-class women with similar 'provoking agents'. One in 3 working-class women with a provoking agent went on to experience clinical depression, whilst 1 in 12 middle-class women with a provoking agent went on to do so. Brown and Harris identified the following factors that they believed increased a woman's vulnerability to developing clinical depression:

- The woman losing her mother before 11 years of age;
- Three or more children aged 14 or under living at home;
- Lack of employment outside of the home.

Brown and Harris concluded that:

> Basically we have seen loss events as the deprivation of sources of value or reward. We now go further to suggest that what is important about such loss for the genesis of depression is that it leads to an inability to hold good thoughts about ourselves, our lives and those close to us.
> *(Brown and Harris, 1976, p. 233)*

Unfortunately, for many women, childcare can lead directly to the very situation they describe.

In a later study, Whiffen (1988) found that vulnerability to depression was associated with the following:

- Prepartum depression;
- Marital difficulties;
- Life event stress.

Whiffen also reported that not all women so exposed become depressed and that depressed women were more likely to perceive their baby in terms of his or her being 'difficult' for various reasons.

Cutrona and Troutman (1986) and Pitt (1968) also note that maternal depression is related to maternal perceptions of the baby as 'difficult' and to frequent and longer crying episodes in babies. These findings have led some researchers to suggest that women who succumb to depression have difficult babies whose levels of irritability and unpredictability make maternal care taking efforts largely ineffective. In turn, the woman begins to feel increasingly depressed and inadequate when the best of her efforts fail to comfort the child.

However, optimistic prepartum explanations about infants also predict depressive symptom levels, indicating that symptoms may be precipitated by unrealistic expectations regarding infant behaviour. McIntosh (1986), in an interesting paper concerned with the 'blues', found that the occurrence of the blues was strongly related to the lack of previous experience with babies. McIntosh was of the opinion that lack of experience led to additional stress and anxiety and thereby made the experience of the 'blues' more likely. If this is the case, this may explain the relatively common observation that there is a high incidence of the occurrence of the blues among first-time mothers (see, for example, Yalom et al., 1968; Nott et al., 1976; Priest, 1979). Vulnerability to postnatal depression is probably increased both by discrepancies between real and anticipated outcomes of infant behaviour, and by infant behaviour being perceived to be, or actually being, sufficiently difficult to raise maternal doubts over her capacity to mother.

Ussher, in highlighting the discrepancy between cultural representation and maternal experience, indicates that:

> Children themselves may also contribute to women's madness – however inadvertently. The idealised image of glowing Madonna gaining pleasure and fulfilment from her angelic offspring is far removed from the reality of many women's experience.
>
> (Ussher, 1991, p. 258)

Alternatively, Richman (1978) and McBride (1988) indicate that rates of depression in women are highly correlated with actual behavioural disturbances and health problems occurring in children, and Ussher (1991) notes that women who are depressed are more likely to have a child with sleep problems or temper tantrums. However, whether the problems experienced by the child cause the woman to be depressed, or whether the problems experienced by the woman cause problems for the child, is a matter of conjecture. Clearly, the relationship may work either way and the spiral is likely to be downward. However, both Pound *et al.* (1985) and Hunt (1986) indicate that women who report that they have a difficult child often also report crushing feelings of failure to mother. In short, mothers with difficult children perceive the problems, irrespective of the origins, to be a reflection of their own inadequacy rather than a reflection of the difficult nature of the child.

Morsbach and Fulton (1987) conducted an investigation into the relationship between maternal postnatal depression and the crying behaviour of infants and found no relationship between levels of postnatal distress and infant crying. Consequently, they questioned the relationship between postnatal depression on the one hand and infant behaviour on the other. Alternatively, Cohn and Tronick (1983) had previously demonstrated that babies show disturbance and distress when confronted by a simulation of postnatal depression. However, it must be said that the babies in Cohn and Tronick's study were being confronted by a rather unusual state of affairs and this, in itself, may have created disturbance and distress.

Furthermore, Morsbach and Fulton's findings fail to confirm the findings of Field (1984) and Kitzinger (1984). What is interesting about Morsbach and Fulton's findings is that maternal depression does not seem to affect maternal attempts to comfort babies and that mothers, including depressed mothers, have a relatively realistic assessment of the crying behaviour of their babies. Furthermore, their case studies indicated that when babies cried a lot, their mothers knew the reason, for example colic, why this was the case. Consequently, the situation may be one in which prolonged periods of infant distress that the mother can neither alleviate *nor* understand are the source of maternal distress. It would seem reasonable to suggest that this combination of factors would effectively, and presumably quickly, undermine whatever sense of competence any given mother had managed to achieve.

If one baby can be difficult to cope with, two babies may cause greater problems. Thorpe *et al.* (1991) have found that the emotional wellbeing of mothers of twins is poor relative to that of the mothers of singletons. Thorpe *et al.* are of the opinion that this is because of the greater burden of care that twins present. These researchers acknowledged that age spacing of children was also an important factor. They found that mothers of closely spaced singletons and mothers of twins were at significantly greater risk of depression compared with other mothers. Thorpe *et al.* concluded that whilst the problems experienced by mothers of twins and mothers of closely spaced siblings were similar, the simultaneous demands of two children, the difficulties associated with mobility and the additional financial burden fell more heavily upon the mothers of twins and accounted for their greater vulnerability to depression.

Elliot (1983) took the view that, in effect, postnatal depression may be a realistic response to the life event of birth and the stress associated with the role of mother. Elliot was of the opinion that postnatal depression would be particularly likely to occur if any other stress factors, including additional burdens of care, were applied to a woman already vulnerable owing to her experiences of pregnancy and childbirth.

Motherhood and loss

Doyal (1995) has noted that despite the lip service that is frequently paid to motherhood as a social duty, there has been relatively little research conducted upon childcare from a woman's perspective. In a relatively early piece of work, Boulton (1983) attempted to disentangle women's feelings about childcare from both the women's love of their children and the status afforded to motherhood. This is no easy task, and many of our respondents frequently focused on this difficulty in an attempt to separate their depression over motherhood from their love of their children. Take, for example, these comments of a 38-year-old woman suffering clinical depression following the birth of her first child:

> Oh, I can't explain it really, I love the baby but I hate being a mother. Just having to be there for him all of the time – and feeling guilt on the odd occasion I'm not. Guilt, guilt, guilt that's what being a mother means to me, I have no status, nothing and I worry what this [her depression] might do to him... I love him, I really do but...

Boulton (1983) found that, on the issue of childcare as opposed to motherhood or baby love, two-thirds of the women she interviewed found a sense of meaning in looking after their children. However, one third of her sample did not. Of these, 66 per cent of middle-class respondents and 44 per cent of working-class respondents said that they found looking after children to be an irritating and unrewarding experience, and this was their evaluation of what had become their full-time work. The mothers in Boulton's study cited the following reasons for their dissatisfaction:

- High levels of stress associated with having the sole responsibility for a young child;
- Lack of time for oneself due to the demanding nature of caring for a young child;
- Loss of self-identify associated with becoming a mother.

Richardson (1993) raises similar issues and links maternal distress directly to the social context in which mothering occurs. In particular:

> There is the tremendous responsibility associated with looking after a young child which, because it is rarely shared and because society provides only limited support for carers, is less likely to produce feelings of self importance and self worth than it is of anxiety and stress.
>
> *(Richardson, 1993, p. 2)*

Richardson argues that the rewards and pleasure of motherhood will depend on the following factors:

- The impact that motherhood has on the individual woman's identity;
- The woman's feelings concerning temporary or permanent economic dependence;
- The woman's reaction to the potential of motherhood to result in social isolation;
- The impact of being denied social recognition for the work done in the home.

Richardson argues that when one adopts a feminist perspective and looks at the actual conditions in which women do the work of mothering, it becomes likely rather than unlikely that many mothers will feel unhappy and depressed.

Oakley (1979) has also argued that feelings of depression after childbirth are associated with an overwhelming and multifaceted experience of loss. She cites the following losses as examples of the losses associated with becoming a mother:

- The temporary or permanent loss of employment;
- The loss of status, which in Western societies is derived primarily from employment;
- The loss of independence both personal and financial;
- The loss of privacy both during pregnancy (a loss occurring in the public sphere) and after the birth of the child (a loss occurring in the private sphere);

76

- The loss of social support and social networks due to the social isolation resulting from childcare and the employment-related nature of many social networks;
- The loss of the culturally valued idealised and romanticised vision of motherhood.

However, Oakley is of the opinion that the biggest loss of all is the loss of 'self', that is, a loss of personal identity and individuality that becoming a mother may entail for many women. For example, one of Boulton's respondents made the following observations:

> I think that children take away your whole life – your identity really. They are so demanding they take everything from you, then come the evening...
>
> *(Boulton, 1983, p. 96)*

Such a pervasive sense of loss coexists uneasily with the confused and confusing social messages that Western societies transmit concerning motherhood. A woman is frequently left in a position of knowing what she herself *no longer* is, of knowing what being a mother is *not*, but of not knowing how she can realistically become the good mother that most women want, and try so desperately hard, to be.

Rossi (1968) documented these and related difficulties in a relatively early piece of work. Rossi was of the belief that four factors made the transition to parenthood particularly difficult:

- The lack of preparation through participation and observation due to living in an age-stratified society;
- The lack of any realistic training for parenthood during pregnancy;
- The sheer abruptness of a transition that involves one person having the total responsibility for another totally dependent human being;
- The lack of realistic guidelines for successful parenting in general.

A certain lack of realism resulting in role confusion has been noted by a number of researchers. For example, Price (1988) notes that women in the contemporary situation are being actively encouraged to develop their careers, but messages are also given about the importance of staying at home for the purposes of rearing children. With society being so inconsistent, the individual woman who, if all other things were equal, would have extremely difficult access to childcare services is left trying to make sense out of conflicting and confusing messages.

Price (1988) also notes that there is considerable social confusion about the value of children in Western societies. Children are often actively excluded from the public sphere, and therefore any adult who has the care of children is actively excluded with them. Since most adult business is conducted in the public sphere and it is adult business, by and large, that confers prestige, power and economic reward, children and adults who have the care of children are excluded from that too.

It is in this way that women are left to deal with a major social conflict throughout most of their adult lives. Failing to understand the totally incomprehensible messages concerning the social context and social value of mothering can be a major source of discontent in new mothers, leaving them, literally as well as figuratively, at a loss.

Price (1988) makes the comment that, for many women, motherhood leaves them feeling that they have become faceless, nameless non-adults when they have had a child. This becomes particularly problematic because women are led to believe that once they become mothers they enter the world of 'grown-up' women, thereby gaining some acknowledgement and respect for their womanliness. Instead, they are often left feeling like social outcasts living in a twilight world with no way of knowing how long their alienation will last. Given that role and identity have already been identified as problematic, the very lack of substance to what is widely acclaimed to be the 'core of feminine identity' must be frustrating indeed.

As Antonis (1981) has indicated, the 'core of feminine identity' would seem to involve doing socially devalued work in socially isolating conditions. The cultural rewards for this work would seem to be depersonalisation and marginalisation. Perhaps this is the 'core of feminine identity' that the patriarchy had in mind.

Phoenix and Woollett (1991) take these points further and argue that the tasks of mothering are socially prescribed in such a way that ensures that most women are unable to learn what they are, but do learn that they are extremely difficult to do well. For example:

> The social and psychological constructions of normal mothers (with normal being synonymous with good and with ideal) run counter to the reality of motherhood for many mothers. As a consequence many mothers are socially constructed as pathological, and differences between mothers are not adequately studied or written about.
>
> (Phoenix and Woollett, 1991, p. 13)

Alternatively, the society that fails to offer a realistic definition of what mothering is, is extremely efficient in prescribing what it

78

should not be and who should and should not entertain mother-hood as a possibility. Although motherhood is presented as a highly desirable state, the desirability is only present in a socially prescribed form. Phoenix and Woollett argue that normative social constructions of good/normal mothers are usually implicit rather than explicit. However, the underlying ideas are often reflected in any given society's social and family policy. In general terms, social policy still presumes that contemporary 'families' are traditional in both format and philosophy, despite, over a number of years, assid-uously gathering statistics that prove the opposite. As Wicks (1987) has indicated, an important element of such traditional philoso-phies is that women (socially powerful figures that they are) should ensure that they and their children are provided for without resort to public means.

Busfield (1987) argues that the current ideology concerning moth-erhood would indicate the following ideal circumstances under which it should occur:

- That the woman should be between 20 and 40 years of age;
- That the woman should be married, preferably before conception and definitely before the birth;
- That the woman should stay married for the duration of her children's period of childhood;
- That the woman should be willing to cooperate in a gendered division of labour involving the woman taking primary responsibility for the home and the man taking primary responsibility for income maintenance.

Public condemnation tends to be the fate of those who fall outside of this narrow band of 'worthy' candidates for motherhood. For example, gay and lesbian parents, parents who are single, and teenage mothers are not exactly treated kindly by the welfare state. Given the points made in the previous two sections of this chapter, such public censure can do little but further pressurise women who are suffering from additional burdens of care associated with their situation.

Busfield further indicates that women are still under considerable pressure to fulfil themselves in traditional ways, which include motherhood, even if the end result turns out to be distinctly unful-filling from a feminist perspective.

Furthermore, as Faludi (1992) has demonstrated, maternity is one of the key issues over which the media frequently causes moral panics concerning the 'woman question'. Again, the impact of such debates is highly unlikely to be positive upon those mothers who do not 'fit' into the socially acceptable categories of women who may become mothers.

Busfield argues that stress and anxieties are created by this intense social pressure towards conformity to a highly idealised and essentially unobtainable role. According to Busfield, the effect of this intense sociocultural pressure is further intensified by the social isolation associated with childcare that immediately follows on from what may have been 9 months of internal psychological warfare. Since previous identity, control and independence have all been, at least temporarily, lost, the woman is left in an extremely vulnerable psychosocial condition. It is hard, if not impossible, to perform well, but easy, and almost unavoidable, to perform badly

Motherhood and oppression

Nicolson (1986) makes an interesting connection between depression and oppression. Nicolson is of the opinion that the experience of motherhood is essentially oppressive. For example:

Increasing oppression arguably goes hand in hand with motherhood and may increase with each child but there is no systematic research available on women with several children.

(Nicolson, 1986, p. 142)

Nicolson believes that, for some women, depression after childbirth is acceptable because this period of their lives exposes them to the need for a re-evaluation of their roles and a change in their social relationships. Nicolson argues that this is particularly, but not exclusively, important in the case of a first baby. Nicolson further suggests that this period of reflection makes some women aware of their oppression for the first time or at the very least aware of the full extent of it. Nicolson argues that the arrival of baby provides an amplification, or realisation, of a set of oppressive circumstances or relationships.

Utilising the concept of oppression rather than depression, Chodorow and Contrattos (1982) have argued that the cultural fantasy of the perfect mother has resulted directly in the cultural oppression of women. This cultural oppression is undertaken, according to Chodorow and Contrattos, in the interests of the perfect child, whose needs are also fantasised. Unfortunately, the sad reality of the situation would seem to be, given that it is by and large women who have the care of children, it is simply impossible to be 'anti' woman *and* 'pro' child.

Nicolson (1986) further expands upon the relationship between cultural oppression and depression. She argues that our current reliance on objective measures, correlations and the use of postnatal depression as a diagnostic label indicative of an 'abnormal' mental state has effectively removed any awareness of the sheer extent of the oppression that is part and parcel of both being a woman and becoming a mother. Through a series of interviews conducted with women following childbirth, Nicolson concluded that many women are simply quite naturally reacting to the anxieties and problems that surround this particular time of their lives. Some support for Nicolson's points may be drawn from the observations of Doyal (1995). Doyal notes that depression (an 'illness') is often directly associated with a group's cultural marginalisation (an oppression).

Ussher (1991) takes a particularly strong line on this point and follows earlier labelling theorists (for example, Laing, 1971; Szasz, 1971; Brooks 1973). These theorists argue that the role psychiatry and psychology play in legitimating societal oppression is by no means a minor one. From this perspective, the entire concept of treating, or attempting to treat, the results of oppression as an illness obscures any understanding of the impossible nature of the lives women are forced to live by the norms of the society they live in. Specifically:

> Within the feminist analysis, the labelling process is seen to serve the function of maintaining women's position as outsiders within patriarchal society; of dismissing women's anger as illness – and exonerating the male oppressors; and of dismissing women's misery as the result of some internal flow and thus protecting the misogynistic social structures from any critical gaze. The early dissenters may have been correct in pointing out that psychiatric labels serve society. What they omitted from their analysis was that it is a patriarchal society.
>
> *(Ussher, 1991, p. 167)*

From Ussher's perspective, postnatal depression is a label that serves the patriarchy. Postnatal distress from this perspective is the result of anger coupled with relative powerlessness over the relentlessly brutal forces of the patriarchal oppression of both women and their children.

Conclusion

This chapter has been concerned with the social context of maternal depression and distress. Part one of the chapter was concerned with the relationship between distress and depression. It was shown how distress during the last trimester of pregnancy and the early months of childbearing are extremely common experiences. However, it was also shown that these experiences rarely result in mothers reporting their distress.

The second part of the chapter was concerned with additional burdens of care associated with the social context within which pregnancy and childbirth occurred. It was suggested that pregnancy and childbirth were extremely stressful psychosocial transitions in themselves, and furthermore, suggested that any additional stressor would greatly add to an individual woman's propensity towards experiencing distress and/or depression.

The third part of the chapter was concerned with the overwhelming feeling of loss that has been associated with the successful bearing of children. It was argued that, whilst the woman was left feeling different and irrevocably changed, exactly *what* it was she was supposed to change into was, in cultural terms, blurred and somewhat intangible. Given that childbirth in certain psychological terms is alleged to represent the 'core of feminine identity', it would appear to be the case that the 'core' of this particular experience was frequently felt to be something more akin to a black hole into which one fell into rather than a self-affirmatory experience that one grew out of. It was also suggested that the cultural proscriptions and prescriptions regarding which women might be considered eligible to become mothers did little more than add to the distress of what appears to be an inherently distressing situation for many women.

The final part of the chapter was concerned with the relationship between oppression and depression. It was suggested that a certain amount of maternal distress may be associated with an understanding of the extent to which women are systematically oppressed under the patriarchy. The role of labelling theory was addressed in this final part of the chapter and the extent to which postnatal depression might be considered in terms of an entirely explicable reaction to the oppression of the patriarchy was documented here. Overall, it would seem to be the case, at least in Western societies, that pregnancy and childbirth are commonly undergone but widely unacknowledged psychosocial transitions, at least in cultural terms. Furthermore, these psychosocial transitions are associated with relatively high degrees of distress occurring amongst those who undergo them. The ways in which these transitions are handled by other societies and the possible reasons for the sociocultural invisibility of the psychosocial transitions associated with pregnancy and childbirth that typically occur in Western societies will be the subject of Chapter 5.

References

Antonis, B. (1981) 'Motherhood and Mothering.' In Cambridge University Women's Study Group (eds) *Women in Society: Interdisciplinary Essays.* (London: Virago).

Boulton, M. (1983) *On Being A Mother* (London: Tavistock).

Brooks, K. 'Freudianism is not a basis for Marxist Psychology.' In Brown, P. (ed.) *Radical Psychology* (London: Tavistock).

Brown, T. and Harris, G. (1978) *The Social Origins of Depression* (London: Tavistock).

Busfield, J. (1987) 'Parenting and Parenthood.' In Cohen, G. (ed.) *Social Change and The Life Course* (London: Tavistock).

Cartwright, A. (1988) 'Unintended Pregnancies that lead to Babies.' *Social Science and Medicine* **27**(3): 249–54.

Chodorow, N. and Contrattos, S. (1982)' The Fantasy of the Perfect Mother.' In Thorne, B. and Yalom, M. (eds) *Rethinking the Family: Some Feminist Questions* (New York: Longman).

Cohn, J. F. and Tronik, E. Z. (1983)' Three Month Old Infants' Reactions to Simulated Maternal Depression.' *Child Development* **54**: 185–93.

Cutrona, C.E. and Troutman, B. R. (1986) 'Social Support, Infant Temperament and Parenting Self Efficacy. A Mediational Model of Postpartum Depression.' *Child Development* **57**: 1507–18.

Doyal, L. (1995) *What Makes Women Sick* (London: Macmillan).

Elliot, S. (1983) 'Mood Change during Pregnancy and after the Birth of a Child.' *British Journal of Clinical Psychology* **22**: 295–308.

Faludi, S. (1992) *Backlash* (London: Vintage).

Field, T. M. (1984) 'Early Interactions between Infants and their Postpartum Depressed Mothers.' *Infant Behaviour and Development* **7**: 517–22.

Hunt, H. (1986) 'Women's Private Distress, a Public Health Issue.' *Medicine in Society* **12**: 2.

Kitzinger, S. (1984) *The Experience of Childbirth* (Middlesex: Pelican).

Laing, R. D. (1971) *The Divided Self: An Existential Study in Sanity and Madness* (Harmondsworth: Penguin).

Macarthur, P. (1991) *Women's Health after Childbirth* (University of Birmingham: HMSO).

McBride, A. (1988) *Women's Mental Health Research Agenda. Multiple Roles.* Women's Mental Health Occasional Paper Series. (Rockville MD: National Institute of Mental Health).

McIntosh, J. (1989) 'Models of Childbirth and Social Class. A Study of 80 Working Class Primips.' In Robinson, S. and Thomson, A. (eds) *Midwifery, Research and Childbirth* (London: Chapman and Hall).

Morsbach, G. and Fulton, E. (1987) 'An Investigation into the Relationship between Maternal Postnatal Depression and Crying Behaviour by Infants.' *Maternal and Child Health* August: 244–6.

Nicolson, P. (1986) 'Developing a Feminist Approach to Depression following Childbirth.' In Wilkinson, S. (ed.) *Feminist Social Psychology* (Milton Keynes: Open University Press).

Nott, P. N., Franklin, M., Armitage, C. *et al.* (1976) 'Hormonal Changes and Mood in the Puerperium.' *British Journal of Psychiatry* **128**: 379–83.

Oakley, A. (1979) *Becoming a Mother* (Oxford: Martin Robinson).

Oakley, A. and Chamberlain, G. (1981) 'Medical and Social Factors in Postpartum Depression.' *Journal of Obstetrics and Gynaecology* **1**: 181–7.

O'Hara, M. W. and Zekoski, E. M. (1988) 'Postpartum Depression: A Comprehensive Review.' In Kumar, R. and Brockington, I. F. (eds) *Motherhood and Mental Illness* (London: Wright).

O'Hara, M. W., Nuenaber, D. and Zekoski, E. M. (1984) 'Prospective Study of Postpartum Depression: Prevalence, Course and Predictive Factors.' *Journal of Abnormal Psychology* **93**: 158–71.

O'Hara, M. W., Rehm, L. P. and Campbell, S. B. (1982) 'Predicting Depressive Symptomatology: Cognitive Behavioural Models and Postpartum Depression.' *Journal of Abnormal Psychology* **91**: 457–61.

O'Hara, M. W., Zekoski, E. M., Phillips, L. H. and Wright, E. J. (1990) 'Controlled Prospective Study of Postpartum Mood Disorders: A Comparison of Childbearing and Non-childbearing Women.' *Journal of Abnormal Psychology* **99**(1):3–15.

Phoenix, A., Woollett, A. and Lloyd, E. (1991) *Motherhood, Meanings, Practices and Ideology* (London: Sage).

Pitt, B. (1968) 'Atypical Depression following Childbirth.' *British Journal of Psychiatry* **114**: 1325–35.

Pound, A. (1985) 'The Impact of Maternal Depression on Young Children.' In Stevenson, J. E. (ed.) *Recent Research in Developmental Pathology* (Oxford: Pergamon Press).

Price, J. (1988) *Motherhood and What It Does To Your Mind* (London: Pandora).

Priest, R. (1979) 'Puerperal Depression and its Treatment.' *Journal of Maternal and Child Health* August: 312–7.

Richardson, D. (1990) *Women, Motherhood and Childbearing* (London: Macmillan).

Richman, N. (1978) 'Depression in Mothers of Young Children.' *British Medical Journal* 288

Romito, P. (1990) 'Postpartum Depression and the Experience of Motherhood.' *Acta Obstetricia and Gynaecologica Scandinavia Suppl.* **69**(154): 1–37.

Romito, P. (1993) Work and Health in Mothers of Young Children. Proceedings of the conference on women, health and work. CAPS, Barcelona 11–12 November.

Romito, P. and Zalateo, C. (1992) 'Social History of a Research Project: A Study of Early Postpartum Discharge.' *Social Science and Medicine* **34**(3): 227–35.

Rossi, A. (1968) 'Transition to Parenthood.' *Journal of Marriage and the Family* **30**: 26–39.

Spitzer, R. L., Endicott, J. and Robins, E. (1978) 'Research Diagnostic Criteria: Rationale and Reliability.' *Archives of General Psychiatry* **35**: 773–82.

Stein, A., Cooper, P. J., Dat, A., Campbell, E. and Altham, P. (1989) 'Social Adversity and Perinatal Complications: Their Relation to Postnatal Depression.' *British Medical Journal* **298**: 1073–4.

Stevens, P. and Meleis, A. (1991) 'Maternal Role of Clerical Workers: A Feminist Analysis.' *Social Science and Medicine* **32**(12): 1425–33.

Szasz, T. (1971) *The Manufacture of Madness: A Comprehensive Study of the Inquisition and the Mental Health Movement* (London: Routledge).

Thorpe, K., Golding, J. and Magillivary, I. (1991) 'Comparison of the Prevalence of Depression in Mothers of Twins and Singletons.' *British Medical Journal* **302**(678): 875–8.

Ussher, J. M. (1991) *Women's Madness: Misogyny or Mental Illness* (London: Harvester/Wheatsheaf).

Whiffen, V. E. (1988) 'Vulnerability to Postnatal Depression: A Prospective Multivariate Study.' *Journal of Abnormal Psychology* **97**: 467–74.

Wicks, M. (1987) 'Family Matters and Public Policy.' In Loney, M. (ed.) *The State of the Market: Politics and Welfare in Contemporary Britain* (London: Sage).

Yalom, I. D., Lunde, D. J., Moor, H. and Hamberg, B. A. (1968) 'Postpartum Blues Syndrome: A Description and Related Variables.' *Archives of General Psychiatry* **18**: 16–27.

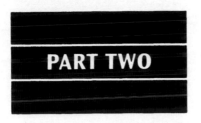

PART TWO

WOMEN'S EXPERIENCES AND INCIDENTS ASSOCIATED WITH DISTRESS AND DEPRESSION FOLLOWING CHILDBIRTH

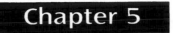

Chapter 5

Childbirth as a Rite of Passage: the Myth of Madonna

Or she may go on trying to fit herself into the order of the world and thereby consign herself forever to the bondage of some stereotype of normal feminity... a perversion if you will.

(Kaplan, 1993, p. 528)

This chapter is concerned with the extent to which postnatal depression and maternal distress may be regarded as occurring cross-culturally. Consequently, the first part of the chapter will be concerned with an evaluation of cross-cultural evidence concerning maternal depression and distress. The role of ritualised expressions relating to the mother's new social status in the immediate post-partum period will be considered here. The role played by the mobilisation of appropriate social support will also be discussed.

The second part of the chapter is concerned with the 'rites of passage' and rituals associated with childbirth in contemporary societies. Anthropological and sociological evidence concerning labour ward 'culture' will be presented here.

The third and final part of the chapter is concerned with Western societies' idealisation of motherhood. The consequences of such an idealisation in terms of distress and/or depression will be addressed. The chapter concludes with a discussion of the complex and multifaceted meanings associated with pregnancy and childbirth in contemporary societies.

Cross-cultural evidence concerning postnatal depression and maternal distress: ritual acknowledgement of status change and social support

Stern and Kruckman (1983) have suggested that an anthropological perspective, incorporating symbolic behaviour and biological approaches, may more effectively illuminate the originals of postnatal depression and maternal distress than either biological or psychosocial research. According to Stern and Kruckman, the anthropological literature provides little evidence of the occurrence of postnatal depression outside Western societies.

However, an absence of evidence may occur for a number of reasons. Specifically, anthropologists may have paid relatively little attention to the issue in their studies of various societies. Alternatively, most anthropological studies rely upon ethnographic field observations, and lack of formal diagnostic testing may result in maternal distress going unreported and consequently unrecorded. Furthermore, cross-cultural comparisons and assessments are extremely difficult. Western conceptualisations of depression use behavioural and experiential criteria that may not be relevant in other cultural settings; that is, postnatal depression and maternal distress may take different forms in different cultures.

Nevertheless, Stern and Kruckman are of the opinion that cultural patterning of the postnatal experience in the societies that anthropologists have studied is the factor that explains the apparently low levels of maternal distress and/or depression. Alternatively, the absence of any cultural patterning of the postnatal period in Western societies is associated with the higher levels of maternal distress and/or depression reported by women. The cultural patterning of a distinct postnatal period involves the following factors:

- Various protective measures designed to reflect the vulnerability of the new mother;
- A period of social seclusion for new mothers;
- A period of mandatory rest for mothers;
- The provision of practical support with domestic tasks. This support is typically provided by female relatives and/or midwives;
- The ritualised social recognition of new mothers' change of social status.

Stern and Kruckman believe that the medicalisation of pregnancy and childbirth in Western societies has led to a lack of social structuring and associated mobilisation of social support during the post-natal period. They associate this lack of structure with the relatively high rates of postnatal depression and maternal distress that occur in such societies.

Pillsbury (1978) came to a similar conclusion when she considered the value of 'doing the month' for Chinese women after childbirth. Traditional custom in China stipulates that a woman should be confined to her home for 1 full month of convalescence after giving birth. During the 'month' the following proscriptions and prescriptions apply:

- Do not wash self or hair and avoid cold water.
- Do not go outside.
- Do not eat raw or cold food.
- Do eat chicken.
- Do not walk or move around.
- Do not go into other people's homes.
- Do not become ill.
- Do not read or cry.
- Refrain from sexual intercourse.
- Do not eat with other members of the family.
- Do not burn incense.

Pillsbury concludes the following:

> This extra attention their families and social networks show them while doing the month seems, in fact, to preclude Chinese women from experiencing post partum depression as understood and taken for granted by Americans – despite the fact that the same biological factors are operative for women of both cultural backgrounds. Neither the Chinese translation of the term 'postpartum depression' nor the concept itself makes much sense to the majority of my informants.
>
> (Pillsbury, 1978, p. 18)

In short, the ritual structuring of the postnatal period is associated with low levels of maternal distress and/or depression following childbirth. However, it must be said that ritual structuring in any society tends to reflect the values of the society. Consequently, the extent to which the values of the individual and the values of the society are similar is a key issue. Furthermore, it has been argued that ritualistic aspects surrounding childbirth are common in Western societies. However, these ritualistic practices are usually cited in connection with their unhelpfulness rather than their helpfulness in connection with the transition to motherhood.

Childbirth as a rite of passage

Van-Gennep's (1960) contribution to our contemporary understanding of the concept of rites of passage has been considerable.
However, this work was written at the turn of the century and translated into English in 1960. Van-Gennep was concerned primarily
with preliterate societies and a wide range of rituals, of which those
associated with birth were only one, albeit important, subset. The
thesis is deceptively simple and states that all rituals involving
passage from one state to another share a single tripartite structure of
rites. The first series of rites involve separation. These rites serve to
separate the individual or group from their previously held social
status or position. The second series of rites are concerned with transition. During the rites of transition, the individual or group is
between social states and is often physically or symbolically excluded
from the society. The third and final series of rites are those of incorporation. These are the rites by which the individual or group is
incorporated into the new social state or position. Van-Gennep was of
the belief that this general structure was adhered to in most societies
and was related to the social necessity of recruiting people who are
born, develop, grow old and die into fixed and relatively unchanging
social systems. In short, rites of passage are necessary because societies outlive their individual members.

Van-Gennep was concerned mainly with societies rather than individuals and claimed that rites of passage eased transitions for societies rather than for individual passengers. However, the theme of
transition associated with rites of passage has been investigated inde-
pendently by Turner (1969). According to Turner, a long transitional
period may be, in certain circumstances, beneficial to the passengers
of some rites. Turner argued that the transitional phase is one in
which people are 'betwixt and between' social states. Therefore
people meet as true equals, and social considerations of status, power
and worth do not apply. Consequently, long periods of transition may
be times of respite and communality.

It is tempting to apply the observations of both Van-Gennep and
Turner to contemporary Western societies' 'management' of childbirth and labour. For example, Homans attempts such an analysis
with the provision that:

> an analysis of pregnancy and birth as a rite of passage is only useful if it
> incorporates into the analysis the viewpoint of the woman concerned. To

become a mother has different meanings to women in industrial society, depending on their social class and ethnic background.

(Homans, 1982, p. 260)

For example, the expectations of women, of themselves and of others may be very different, both across and within cultures. Consequently, their experiences of pregnancy and childbirth are likely to be varied. Some specific examples, derived from practice, are:

- Women for whom English is a second language and whose relatives may be in another country;
- Women who are refugees and who have been displaced in mid-pregnancy;
- Women who expect, or who are expected, to produce a baby of a particular sex and who do not;
- Women who aspire to a career and who find themselves expected to stay at home following childbirth;
- Women who aspire to a certain experience of childbirth and whose experience differs from their expectations.

This is precisely the problem with attempting to utilise the concept of rites of passage in contemporary Western societies. Specifically, for a rite of passage to ease the transition for passengers, the passengers have to believe in the efficacy of the ritual. Where belief systems differ, problems are likely to be encountered. This is well documented by Jones and Dougherty (1982) who argue, in the same volume as Homans, that the elements of rites of passage are clearly present in births occurring in hospitals in contemporary Western societies. However, it is argued that the homogenous 'management' of childbirth and labour coexists uneasily with the heterogeneous customs and attitudes of pregnant women.

Jones and Dougherty utilise Van-Gennep's concept of the tripartite structure of rites of passage in order to illustrate the applicability of this concept to contemporary Western 'rituals'. Specifically, they describe the ways in which women, once their pregnancy has advanced are encouraged to withdraw from social activities and appearances in public as an example of rites of separation:

They have the effect of reducing the need for her to meet the demands of her previous role as money earner, daughter, autonomous individual and even as wife.

(Jones and Dougherty, 1982, p. 279)

According to Jones and Dougherty, hospitalisation dominates the stage of transition that is hidden from the wider society. The stage of transition is further characterised by the depersonalisation and enforced passivity of the pregnant and/or labouring woman:

> She is physically inspected mainly in the area of her genitals. She is expected to remain lying down and, at inspections, near delivery and afterwards, her legs are in straps which retain them in a raised and apart position.
>
> *(Jones and Dougherty, 1982, p. 280)*

According to Jones and Dougherty, women in this position may experience the situation in which they find themselves in one of two ways. Women who are experiencing 'good' births feel excited and women who experience 'bad' births are mortified. The 'good' or 'bad' motives of those who would put another human being in such a position are not commented on by the authors.

Rites of reincorporation take place on the postnatal ward as the woman enters into relationships with others who have undergone a similar transition and the woman begins to become a mother. Eventually, rites of reincorporation are completed when the woman is discharged from hospital and reincorporated into her own home with her new baby.

The value of Jones and Dougherty's work lies in their identification of the apparent enactment of a relatively primitive ritual process upon a heterogeneous group of women passengers. Presumably, the extent to which any individual woman might interpret her experiences as 'good' ones would depend upon the extent to which she accepted the belief systems inherent in this process. It might be argued that the medical model of the 'management' of childbirth and labour carries within it a primitive system of beliefs and practices that may be at best irrelevant and at worst damaging to women with different complex belief systems.

Cheal (1988) has done much to clarify the relatively complex role that rituals play in contemporary and largely secular societies. Cheal identified three types of ritual relevant to such societies:

- Rituals of reification (associated with the past);
- Rituals of resource management (associated with the present);
- Rituals of reproduction (associated with the future).

According to Cheal, rituals of reification:

are believed to have their origins in traditions inherited from the past, which cannot be changed because the flow of time cannot be reversed. These rituals of reification have most useful effects in maintaining boundaries and internal solidarity of social groups, and they have a conservative social influence. They are therefore particularly highly valued by people whose position and authority depends upon maintaining the integrity of existing social structures.

(Cheal, 1988, p. 283)

It is tempting to apply Cheal's notion of rituals of reification to the medical model of childbirth and labour, which, whilst clearly unacceptable to some women, certainly protects both the position and the authority of the medical profession.

Alternatively, rituals of resource management share many similarities with rites of passage:

Rituals of resource management celebrate success in 'doing something' about the situation through rational use of available resources. The origin of these rituals is in the present which is experienced as a boundary between the limitations of the past and the proposals for a better future.

(Cheal, 1988, p. 284)

Specifically, doing something about a transition is argued by Cheal to be a matter of sociocultural importance. It is tempting to apply this notion to women who expect to be actively involved in planning their care during pregnancy and childbirth, that is, they wish to secure, given available resources, the best transition and best future, however that might be defined, for themselves and their baby.

However, the importance of rituals of resource management in contemporary Western societies may reflect a masculine perspective. Whilst Cheal presents his work in gender-neutral terms, MacSween (1995) persuasively argues that gender neutrality is fundamentally masculine:

In our equal opportunities cultures a non-gendered subjectivity is – formally at least – 'available' for women, who are simultaneously non-gendered subjects and feminine objects. The superficial gender neutrality of individuality masks its fundamentally masculine character. The social construction of masculine and feminine around difference means that being a man is 'not being a woman'; being a woman is 'not being a man'. Women who aspire to 'non-gendered' subjectivity undercut this structure of difference but rarely perceive it directly.

(MacSween, 1995, p. 93)

MacSween suggests that the aspirations of middle-class women towards gender neutrality play a central part in the development of anorexia nervosa, which, typically, affects adolescent girls at puberty. MacSween contends that anorexia represents one of the many individual solutions to the cultural contradictions associated with gender-neutral success and feminine identity. Since childbirth is another transition associated with the achievement of 'true femininity', it would seem reasonable to suggest that these cultural contradictions may exert their effects, albeit in a different context.

The final group of rituals identified by Cheal are those of reproduction. These rituals are derived from representations of the end and serve to protect the present by promising a continuing social future. Cheal is of the belief that the fear of premature endings, in the absence of new beginnings, actively fuels rituals of reproduction in contemporary societies. Interestingly enough, it is precisely the lack of rituals of reproduction in the postpartum period which Stern and Kruckman associate with high rates of maternal distress and depression in contemporary Western societies. The observations made in Chapter 4 would seem to indicate that many women experience motherhood as a 'black hole' into which they fall rather than an exhilarating and exciting experience with a new baby. In the words of one of our respondents, a 32-year-old mother, upon the birth of her first child:

I don't know. I just felt that my life was over somehow. That, that was it, there was nothing else really.

Consequently, it is difficult to disagree with Stern and Kruckman's observations concerning contemporary Western societies, that is, that the lack of structural appreciation of the daunting and demanding experiences of motherhood in the early postpartum period probably contribute to maternal experiences of distress and may, in certain instances, lead to postnatal depression. Interestingly enough, it is these very points which are now being discussed in the relevant medical literature (see, for example, O'Hara et al., 1990)

In a study that looks at the culture of the labour ward, Green et al. (1990) looked at prevalent stereotypes of childbearing women and tested their accuracy, in terms of the likelihood of the development of postnatal depression. In connection with these two stereotypes of childbearing women, Green et al. argue that these, albeit crude, stereotypes of pregnant women are important in as much as they are frequently used to justify the ways in which maternity services should or should not operate. For example:

It is not widely appreciated that pregnant women are not only emotionally unstable, they are intensely egocentric... in this egocentric state, encouragement to participate can result in a fierce demand to dictate.

(Francis, 1985, p. 69)

According to Green *et al.* (1986), two of the most common stereotypes that affect maternity services provision are the 'well educated middle class NCT type' and the 'uneducated working class woman'. The 'negative' characteristics of the 'well educated NCT type' are as follows:

- A woman who holds fixed and inflexible ideas about choice and control in childbirth;
- A woman who holds overly high expectations of childbirth as a fulfilling personal experience;
- A woman who is therefore likely to be disappointed and at risk of developing postnatal depression;
- A woman who holds a rigid, intellectual approach to labour and therefore may be unable to 'let go' and may inhibit her contractions;
- A woman who is giving birth to her first child;
- A woman who is focused upon childbirth as an experience in itself, possibly to the exclusion of the wellbeing of her baby.

A more positive reading of this 'labour ward' stereotype is:

- The woman is well informed, reasonable and rational.
- The woman attends childbirth preparation classes.
- The woman wishes to be involved in the decision-making processes and to communicate on an equal basis with staff.
- The woman is willing to adapt to changing circumstances should the need to do so arise.
- The woman wishes to maintain some degree of control over relevant decision-making processes.
- The woman's goal is ultimately the safe delivery of her baby.

The negative characteristics of the 'uneducated working class woman' are as follows:

- Out of control of her fertility;
- Wilfully ignorant;
- Fails to turn up for antenatal clinic appointments;
- Uninterested in emotional fulfilment;

- Refuses to consider the issues surrounding pain control;
- Abdicates all responsibility to the staff.

Alternatively a more positive assessment of this stereotype may involve:

- Acceptance of expert opinion;
- Does as she is asked;
- Values the end product rather than the process.

Green *et al.* (1990) found considerable support for the positive stereotypical views of most women and found that the women involved in their study were far more complex than the potentially self-protecting stereotypes utilised by health-care professionals. Green *et al.* concluded that:

> Systems of care which allow midwives and mothers to get to know each other (preferably before the birth) could do much to reduce reliance on stereotypes, with beneficial results for all concerned.
>
> *(Green* et al., *1990, p. 131)*

The aims of *Changing Childbirth* (Department of Health, 1993) should, if they are realised, go some way towards solving the problems that Green *et al.* have identified. The major problem would appear to be the inflexible nature of the culture of the labour ward, coupled with, until recently at least, the dominance of the medical model that seeks to impose a particular ideological view of the position of women, often against the views of the women involved. Resistance to such an imposition appears to be associated, in the minds of those who seek to impose it, with 'things going badly' for women who resist.

Unfortunately, stereotypes have a tendency to become self-fulfilling, unless their accuracy is doubted and consequently clarified. Consider, for example, these comments made by a 27-year-old woman about the caesarean delivery of her first child:

> I couldn't believe it afterwards, all of that time and they never said anything because of that [i.e. a belief on the part of the obstetric staff that, despite having a relatively high risk of breech presentation, she wanted to attempt a vaginal delivery]. If I had known, they could have done anything they liked a lot earlier. Why the hell did they let me go through that... the least they could have done is to bloody well ask me what I thought!

In terms of an analysis based upon Van-Gennep's schema of transitions negotiated in 'primitive' societies, it is informative to note how the transition to full femininity is believed to be achieved in complex Western industrial ones:

> She is physically inspected mainly in the area of her genitals. She is expected to remain lying down...
>
> *(Jones and Dougherty, 1982, p. 280)*

This imposition of passivity, coupled with the alleged 'irrationality' of pregnant women, together with the desire for control that seems to dominate themes throughout the obstetric literature quoted throughout this book, would be interpreted by Haste (1994) in terms of the imposition of crude cultural dichotomies that lie at the heart of sociocultural definitions of gender. In particular, Haste argues that femininity is associated with irrationality, passivity and chaos, whilst masculinity is associated with action, rationality and control. Arguably, the culture of the labour ward represents a microcosm of conservative sociocultural attitudes towards femininity, and to achieve 'full femininity', passivity, irrationality and chaos must be imposed if they are not already present.

Furthermore, if undue passivity, irrationality and chaos are present, that too is devalued precisely because it is socioculturally 'feminine'. What is most disturbing about the stereotypes forwarded by Green *et al.* (1990) is the 'no-win' scenario associated with the negative stereotypes they describe. If a woman conforms to sociocultural expectations of femininity, she is devalued, although Green *et al.* do concede that to some she might appear to be the 'perfect patient'. Alternatively, if she does not conform, she is treated as an immature woman who is likely to become a 'management' problem.

Given this analytical framework, the more recent proposals for changing maternity services put forward in *Changing Childbirth* might be said to represent a move away from what Cheal would call rituals of reification towards the, possibly more realistic, rituals of resource management.

Unfortunately, Cheal's conceptualisation of rituals of resource management emphasises actively taking control of, and rationally appraising, a potentially fluid situation. In sociocultural terms, this would be a 'masculine' approach. This tension between sociocultural concerns over masculine versus feminine dichotomies might be said to lie at the heart of debates surrounding *Changing Childbirth*.

In particular, the rejection of the notion of passive labouring and passive mothering by a sizeable proportion of the female population involves a challenge to the predominant cultural norms and values regarding what is appropriate 'feminine' behaviour. In these terms, the issue is much greater than one of individual choice. This in itself may go some way to explaining the heated debates associated with this area. Furthermore, the notion of active control and/or consent would appear to be central to any realistic understanding of birth trauma and to cognitive explanations of postnatal depression. The feminist analyses presented in Chapter 4 are also of relevance. Specifically, active mothering would by necessity be culturally 'invisible' because the active nature of being a mother is at odds with sociocultural views concerning the 'natural' passivity and subservience of women.

Consequently, the passage to 'true feminine identity' in contemporary Western societies exposes a profound sociocultural contradiction that individual women are left to solve for themselves, a

... perversion if you will

(Kaplan, 1993, p. 528)

– and a perversion if you will not?

The idealisation and denigration of motherhood: the myth of Madonna

If, in sociocultural terms, it is accepted that the path to 'true feminine identity' leads inexorably via pregnancy and childbirth towards passivity and subservience, the active responsibility for the total care of a dependant human being then becomes problematic in itself. There should be 'nothing to it', but of course there is.

As Carter (in press) wryly observes, the original 'Madonna' is remembered for her obedience and her passivity. An alternative reading might suggest a brave woman who was willing to risk becoming a single parent in first-century Palestine because of her unshakeable convictions. However, this is not the 'Madonna' who is remembered.

Welldon (1992) is also highly critical of the crude 'Madonna'– 'Whore' dichotomy that she believes to be responsible for the idealisation and denigration of motherhood in contemporary Western societies. Welldon observes that one of the central paradoxes surrounding motherhood is that, whilst in sociocultural terms women are expected to be both passive and powerless, they are also expected by society to:

> behave as if they had been provided with magic wands which not only free them from previous conflicts, but also equip them to deal with the new emergencies of motherhood with skill, precision and dexterity.
>
> *(Welldon, 1992, p. 18)*

Welldon goes on to suggest, that in certain circumstances, unrealistic social expectations may lead to a terrible sense of despair and inadequacy, a point equally well made by Price (1988). However, Welldon argues that this crushing sense of failure may easily turn into feelings of hatred and revenge that are directed towards the new baby.

Stanworth (1994) argues that the 'magic wand' to which Welldon refers is provided by the convenient theory of a universal maternal instinct; that is, women are simply supposed to 'know what to do'. Stanworth is also highly critical concerning women's alleged increasing control over motherhood. Two reasons are offered to support this perspective. Firstly, she argues that the social definition of motherhood has changed and that mothers are now expected to be able to lavish more 'care' (physical, social and intellectual) on their children than at any other point in history. More relevantly, the second reason relates to the powerful ideology of motherhood that holds that it is the natural, desired and ultimate goal of normal women. The power of this socially defined concept of a universal instinct is still, according to Stanworth, used to override women's wishes with regard to childbearing. In short, the concept of a maternal instinct often coexists uneasily with obstacles to autonomous motherhood. According to the ideologies, all women want children, but women who are not in a permanent relationship with a man are expected to curtail their 'instincts', presumably in the interests of the child. The importance of the notion of 'instinct' is that, by 'nature', to act on instinct is irrational, potentially chaotic and uncontrollable – socioculturally 'feminine' in Haste's (1994) terms.

O'Brien (1983) has suggested that the masculine sense of disconnectedness from pregnancy has underpinned cultural patterns that not only subdue women, but also give men an illusion of procreative continuity and power. However, the power that men are attempting to usurp is ultimately biologically defined, and the assumption that all women stand, or should do, in the same relationship to biological potential for reproduction is questionable. It has been argued throughout this chapter that different women take different views of pregnancy and childbirth. If this were not the case, the variations in expectations and experiences would not have been so widely documented. However, for women to live or attempt to live by the 'myth of Madonna' is argued by some authors, notably Welldon (1992) and Kaplan (1993), to be ultimately destructive to both the woman and her child. Kaplan is particularly concerned with contemporary cultural theories that purport to acknowledge women's active sexuality but in fact restrict the notion of femininity within the narrow confines not of motherhood, but of active heterosexuality. In the case of abuse of children she argues that:

> a mother does not abuse her children for want of a phallus but out of conviction that she is nothing at all without a powerful phallic-being in her life and out of the rage engendered by this idealization. When the conditions of family life are such that a woman has no other choice but to achieve her own personal salvation through her children or through her husband or her lover, that's when the violence [the inter- and intrapersonal violence that Kaplan identifies from her clinical practice] begins.
>
> *(Kaplan, 1993, p. 411)*

Clearly, subscribing or attempting to subscribe to the myth of Madonna may be associated with both women and children paying a relatively high price for their conformity.

Conclusion

This chapter has been concerned with the extent to which postnatal depression and maternal distress manifest themselves cross-culturally. Issues pertinent to comparative analysis and relevant cross-cultural evidence were presented in the first part of the chapter. It was suggested that, in relatively homogenous societies, the ritualisation of pregnancy and childbirth may provide a valuable vehicle for the receipt of social support for women recently delivered of children. In turn, this support may help to alleviate postpartum distress and depression. It was further suggested that social support for mothers in Western, industrial societies is somewhat lacking.

The second part of the chapter looked at ritualistic aspects of pregnancy and childbirth in complex industrial societies. The assumption that rituals necessarily facilitate transitions for passengers of rites was evaluated. It was suggested that, although ritual elements were present within the medical model of the management of childbirth, such elements effectively disempowered many women owing to the heterogeneous expectations concerning maternity held by women. In short, the imposition ritualised or otherwise of the 'one right way' to approach childbirth is inappropriate in complex, largely secular cultures. Alternative conceptualisations of ritual were introduced and found, at least in theory, to offer greater flexibility in terms of individual support.

The final part of the chapter was concerned with the relationship between the assumptions lying behind the medical model of childbirth and the culture from which they arose. It was suggested that the medical model of childbirth merely reflected broader sociocultural issues concerning the appropriate role of women in society. It was argued that, in many ways, such assumptions were at best overtly simplistic and at worst damaging to women and children. It may be further suggested that labour and childrearing are approached in a multitude of different ways by a multitude of different women. Unfortunately, sociocultural attitudes fail to reflect the varied nature of the experiences of mothering and may, therefore, be said to be associated with a certain degree of maternal distress and/or outright anger. Consequently, it is concluded that maternal choice and control are issues central to childbirth and childrearing. Resorting to the use of primitive devices or formulae associated with ritualisation and the widespread use of stereotypes is likely to provide an inadequate framework within which to understand pregnancy and childbirth.

If the meaning of pregnancy and childbirth is complicated in advanced industrial societies, it follows that the meaning of postnatal depression and maternal distress is equally complicated.

Attempts to understand the complex and multifaceted nature of women's experiences of postnatal depression are the subject of Chapter 6.

References

Carter, N. (in press) 'Behind the Icon: Distorted Images and Social Control.' In Littlewood, J. (ed.) *Misconstruing the Feminine: Social Change and Social Control* (London: Macmillan).

Cheal, D. (1988) 'The Post-modern Origin of Ritual.' *Journal for the Theory of Social Behaviour* **18**(3): 269–90.

Department of Health (1993) *Changing Childbirth* The Report of the Expert Maternity Group (London: HMSO).

Francis, H. H. (1985) 'Obstetrics: A Consumer Orientated Service? The Case Against.' *Maternal and Child Health* **10**: 69–72.

Green, J. M., Kitzinger, J. V. and Coupland, V. A. (1986) 'The Division of Labour: Implications of Medical Staffing Structure for Doctors and Midwives on the Labour Ward.' *Child Care and Development Group* (Cambridge: University of Cambridge).

Green, J. M., Kitzinger, J. V. and Coupland, V. A. (1990) 'Stereotypes of Childbearing Women: A Look at Some Evidence' *Midwifery* **6**: 125–32.

Haste, H. (1994) *The Sexual Metaphor* (Hemel Hempstead: Harvester/ Wheatsheaf).

Homans, H. (1982) 'Pregnancy and Birth as Rites of Passage for Two Groups of Women in Britain.' In MacCormack C. P. (ed.) *Ethnography of Fertility and Birth* (London: Academic Press).

Jones, A. D. and Dougherty, C. (1982) 'Childbirth in a Scientific and Industrial Society.' In MacCormack, C. P. (ed.) *Ethnography of Fertility and Birth* (London: Academic Press).

Kaplan, L. J. (1993) *Female Perversions: The Temptations of Madame Bovary* (London: Penguin).

MacSween, M. (1995) *Anorexic Bodies: A Feminist and Sociological Perspective on Anorexia Nervosa* (London: Routledge).

O'Brien, M. (1983) *The Politics of Reproduction* (London: Routledge and Kegan Paul).

O'Hara, M. W., Zekoski, E. M., Philips, L. H. and Wright, E. J. (1990) 'Controlled Prospective Study of Postpartum Mood Disorders: Comparison of Childbearing and Non-childbearing Women.' *Journal of Abnormal Psychology* **99**(1): 3–15.

Pillsbury, B. L. K. (1978) 'Doing the Month: Confinement and Convalescence of Chinese Women After Childbirth.' *Social Science and Medicine* **12**: 11–22.

Price, J. (1988) *Motherhood: What it Does to your Mind* (London: Pandora).

Stanworth, M. (1994) 'Reproductive Technologies and the Deconstruction of Motherhood.' In *The Polity Reader in Gender Studies* (Cambridge: Polity Press).

Stern, G. and Kruckman, L. (1983) 'Multi-Disciplinary Perspectives on Post-Partum Depression: An Anthropological Critique.' *Social Science and Medicine* **17**(15): 1027–41.

Turner, V. (1969) *The Ritual Process* (Chicago: Aldine).

Van-Gennep, A. (1960) *The Rites of Passage* (Chicago: University of Chicago Press).

Welldon, E. V. (1992) *Mother, Madonna, Whore: The Idealization and Denigration of Motherhood* (London: Guildford Press).

Chapter 6

Motherhood and the Experience of Distress and Depression

There is a growing recognition for the need to increase general and clinical awareness of postnatal complications. In all the antenatal classes Jean and I attended not one raised the issue of postnatal depression or considered the relationship changes that were bound to occur and how these could be dealt with. All of this shows perhaps, the over medicalisation of childbirth.

(Gilbert, 1992, p. 48)

This chapter is concerned with motherhood and experiences of distress and depression. The first part of the chapter looks at some of the issues surrounding the classification of postnatal depression as a psychiatric disorder in its own right. Part two of the chapter is concerned with the advantages associated with viewing postnatal depression as a discrete medical condition. Part three of the chapter is concerned with the disadvantages of classifying postnatal depression as a medical disorder. Part four of the chapter draws upon the experiences of five women in order to illustrate postnatal depression occurring as a possible consequence of:

- Physical birth trauma;
- Psychological birth trauma;
- The reactivation of negative past experiences;
- Inadequate social support networks;
- Loss of self-identity.

Whilst the overall intention is to illustrate the importance of a specific theme, maternal distress and postnatal depression rarely result from the consequences of one discrete and easily identifiable event. The chapter concludes with a discussion of the trauma and distress that may be associated with giving birth to a healthy baby.

The classification of postnatal depression as a psychiatric disorder

Until recently, postnatal depression was not considered to be a psychiatric disorder that warranted a separate categorisation under the World Health Organization's International Classification of Diseases (ICD 10; World Health Organization, 1992). According to ICD 10, mental disorders that occur around the time of childbirth can only be classified as puerperal if no other classification can be applied.

ICD 10 specifies that a puerperal-related diagnosis must be related only to an illness commencing within the first 6 weeks after birth, where there is not sufficient evidence available to reach an alternative diagnosis or where there are pertinent clinical features that make an alternative diagnosis inappropriate.

Table 6.1   The ICD 10 classification of puerperal disorders

F53	Mental and behavioural disorders with the puerperium not elsewhere classified
	This classification should be used for mental disorders associated with the puerperium (commencing within 6 weeks of delivery) that do not meet the criteria for disorders classified elsewhere in [ICD 10], either because insufficient information is available or because it is considered that special additional clinical features are present which make classification elsewhere inappropriate. It will usually be possible to classify mental disorders associated with the puerperium by using two other codes, the first is from elsewhere in Ch. V (F) and indicates the specific type of mental disorder (usually affective – F30–F39). The second is 099.3 (mental diseases and diseases of the nervous system complicating the puerperium) of ICD 10
F53.0	Mild mental and behavioural disorders associated with the puerperium, not elsewhere classified
	This includes postnatal depression No. 5
F53.1	Severe mental and behavioural disorders associated with the puerperium not elsewhere classified
	Includes puerperal psychosis No. 5
F53.8	Other mental and behavioural disorders associated with the puerperium, not elsewhere classified.
F53.9	Puerperal mental disordered unspecified

Source: World Health Organization (1992).

dilemmas and conflicts in the context of marriage, family relationships, reproduction, child rearing, divorce, ageing, education and work.

(World Health Organization, 1993, p. 3)

Employing the World Health Organization for a frame of reference, could it really be argued that using a medical framework is potentially inaccurate and that the feelings that women experience after childbirth relate to what are considered to be the ordinary and therefore normal circumstances of their lives? Within this context, the issue of postnatal depression as a disorder separate from depression can also be raised. The World Health Organization quote looks at women's lives in a number of contexts and identifies that the dilemmas in these areas often lead to mental health problems. Therefore, would it be possible to argue that the depression following childbirth is not a separate condition but part of a broader picture, with childbirth being one of many triggers that may produce the very real and distressing symptoms that have been identified in postnatal depression?

Russo (1985) has shown that, epidemiologically, there is a link between mental disorder and conditions commonly experienced by women in their lives, that is, alienation, powerlessness and poverty. Again, we can see that these conditions feature in many areas of women's lives and not just around childbirth. However, powerlessness during childbirth (Kitzinger, 1992) has already been noted to be a significant predisposing factor, and Brown and Harris (1978) have written on the significant relationship between poverty and depression in women's lives. O'Hara *et al.* (1990) also observed that the incidence of depression 6 weeks post-delivery was similar to the incidence of depression reported by women who had not been pregnant. O'Hara *et al.* (1990) matched pregnant women with a control group of non-pregnant women. Again, no difference was found in rates of depression between the two groups. This would appear to indicate that even if the parameters of a medical model are considered to be acceptable, there is conflict concerning the correct diagnosis within this area.

This could then lead back to the guidelines of the ICD 10 (see Table 6.1 above), which recognises the diagnosis of postnatal depression only in limited and fairly precise circumstances. As is constantly the case with postnatal depression and maternal distress, it is extremely difficult to develop any firm conclusions. What is certain, however, is that whatever theoretical constructs or frameworks are adopted, the experiences of women who have been affected are very real and extremely trau-

The DSM IV unlike its predecessors, has now included a new specifier with postpartum onset, (Table 6.2) the intention being to reflect evidence that this prognosis and diagnosis have a certain degree of validity.

Table 6.2   Postpartum specifier

1. It can be applied to current or most recent major depressive, manic or mixed episode of major depressive disorder, Bipolar I disorder, Bipolar II disorder or brief psychotic disorder if the onset is within 4 weeks of childbirth

2. The symptomatology of the postpartum disorders does not have to differ from the symptomatology in non postpartum episodes and may include psychotic features

3. Fluctuating course and mood lability may be more common in postpartum episodes

4. When delusions are present they often concern the new-born. In psychotic and non-psychotic ideation, obsessional thoughts, lack of concentration and psychomotor agitation

5. Women with postpartum major depressive episodes often have severe anxiety, panic attacks and spontaneous crying long after the usual duration of the baby blues and insomnia

Source: DSM IV.

Social advantages to viewing postnatal depression as a medical disorder

There are certain sociocultural advantages in viewing psychological disturbances in the puerperium as a medical condition. In particular, the medicalisation of women's experiences gives a readily identifiable method of definition, identification and treatment, without threatening or posing any challenge to the *status quo* or fabric of society.

The most profound message in 'The Yellow Wallpaper'... is the one about how women's problems are constantly individualised: it is the individual woman who has the problem, and, even if many individual women have the same problem, the explanation of a defective psychology rather than of a defective social structure is usually preferred... The medicalisation of unhappiness as depression is one of the greatest disasters of the twentieth century.

(Oakley, 1993, p. 8)

Dealing with unforeseen psychological disturbances at a time when the cultural myth places an emphasis on fulfilment and positive experience is traumatic enough without having to confront the concept of a structurally unequal society. It may be far easier to accept the medicalisation of unhappiness as a culturally acceptable alternative that fits more readily into the framework of society. Take, for example, the following quote from a 25-year-old woman, on her experience after the birth of her first baby:

'You know if they'd told me I'd got postnatal depression it would've been much easier. Like I could get some help. There would be somebody to sort me out'.

So the medical label of postnatal depression can be argued to legitimise women's emotions in a potentially unthreatening way, giving society and the woman a relatively safe option. The medical label is also advantageous for health professionals, as it again allows a system of diagnosis, recognition and treatment. This type of formalised approach fits in well with our current health-care model. It legitimises the existence of the dealers and healers of health, again reinforcing our cultural expectations and acting within the boundaries of our cultural norms. Ussher (1991) argues that in certain ways the experts and professionals need the labels of madness and depression to justify or quantify their existence. Likewise Cox and Holden (1994) write about the uses and advantages of the Edinburgh Postnatal Depression Scale (EPDS), stating that it not only gives a woman 'permission' to speak and a health professional 'permission' to listen, but also gives health professionals a structured approach to the identification of depression and a means of intervention. In addition to being a medical diagnosis, 'depression' is also a commonly used expression. We can talk about feeling depressed but not necessarily need medical intervention.

Depression is a readily available term, although contextually it may mean many different things. It does not challenge our belief systems dramatically; it is possible to find a niche for it in our cognitive scheme of reference.

Depression also fits into what Rubel (1977) identified as a folk illness. Rubel defines folk illnesses or syndromes as something:

from which members of a particular group claim to suffer and for which their culture provides an aetiology, diagnosis, preventative measures and regimes of health.

(Rubel, 1977, p. 251)

Rubel's concept of a folk syndrome is applicable to our society's definition of depression as a common usage term.

Disadvantages of viewing postnatal depression as a medical disorder

Certainly the medicalisation of postnatal depression offers a convenient framework for maternal distress, and it can be argued that to deny its existence as a medical disorder is to be at risk of denying or trivialising the very real and distressing experiences of many women. What needs to be explored is whether postnatal depression is a separate condition and whether there are inherent problems central to a medical frame of reference.

Doyal (1995) argues that although Western medicine gives a powerful framework for the description and classification of individuals' experience of sickness, there are limitations to the framework:

Two aspects of medical practice have come under particular scrutiny: its narrowly biological orientation and its separation of individuals from their wider social environment.

(Doyal, 1995, p. 15)

Doyal argues that the model of medicine as the engineer repairing faulty machinery fails to comprehend the relationship between mind and body and is frequently at risk of separating individuals from their social and cultural realities.

This medicalised approach to women's health and wellbeing can be argued to be a cultural heritage, which may go some way to explaining the acceptability of the medical model. Historically, we have a tradition of women's problems being given a biological focus. This can be argued as an issue relating to the manifestation of the patriarchal control of women's minds, bodies and fertility. In particular, medical science has made connections between women's mental health and their reproductive capacities or incapacities. Showalter (1987) argues that madness is symbolically a female malady even when it occurs in males.

In addition to this, the World Health Organization's view of psychosocial and mental aspects of women's health states that:

Circumstances and conditions that society accepts as normal or ordinary often lead to mental health problems in women. Women fa

matic, and it would be wrong to minimise women's realities by using inappropriate terms of reference and theoretical constructs.

Case histories of the onset of postnatal depression

What follows are five case studies that illustrate:

- Physical birth trauma;
- Psychological birth trauma;
- The reactivation of negative past experiences;
- Inadequate social support networks;
- Loss of self-identity.

Each case history has been chosen to illustrate a specific theme. However, it must be stressed that many issues contribute to a given woman's experience of distress and depression. It is rare indeed for postnatal distress and depression to result from one discrete and easily identifiable event or intervention.

■ CASE HISTORY 1 ■

Consequences of physical birth trauma

This was Paula's first birth experience following 6 years in a stable relationship. When Paula found out she was pregnant, she was 31 years old:

I was thirty-one years old – I felt like a granny in clinic!

Although the pregnancy was planned and both Paula and her partner were pleased about it, neither of them had had any experience of childcare, so had planned to take up parentcraft classes both at the local hospital and with the National Childbirth Trust. However, Paula, in retrospect, felt that the reality of her early parenting experience did not correspond with her expectations:

The reality was totally different. I feel that the first eight months of Jessica's life were a complete nightmare and blur. It was an awful time, that I swore I would never put myself or my family through again. Just thinking back on it makes me start to panic a little. Everything totally fell apart when I was in labour, it was nothing like I'd planned or imagined.

For Paula, everything had been straight forward antenatally. Labour began with mild backache, which felt uncomfortable but bearable. Following her waters breaking, Paula began to contract, so contacted the local hospital:

What a mess – all over the sofa. Not long after that I started to contract and I thought 'this is it, here we go'. I phoned the hospital and they said to come in. I got Steve home from work and we took ourselves off to the hospital. I felt great, really excited, and when we got there the midwife checked us over, all seemed well.

Paula's labour continued to progress well over the following hours, but then things seemed to slow down and she was advised to have a syntocinon infusion sited intravenously to speed labour up again. Paula did not feel so comfortable with the intravenous infusion, her contractions were becoming more difficult to cope with and her mobility had been limited by the use of the infusion and the subsequent continuous fetal monitoring.

I think I must've been on this drip for about two hours, when the midwife got the doctor in again. Jessica's heart beat had dropped down and she was distressed badly. Things happened very rapidly. I was in pain, the drip made the contractions really hurt, and people were rushing around.

At this point Paula was rushed to theatre for an emergency caesarean section, her last memory as she left the room being of Steve in a corner looking very pale and shocked, vomiting.

Nobody explained what was happening, it was all a bit rushed. I really thought I was going to die and that the baby was already dead.

The trauma of Jessica's birth had a deep effect on Paula. She woke up with a blood transfusion, a urinary catheter and a wound drain, and she was in pain and vomiting.

I didn't want her near me or in my room. I didn't believe that the baby was mine at all, or that I'd even had a baby... I felt like my body had been invaded. I didn't even feel as though my body belonged to me anymore. I'd been violated and there was this thing in the cot.

The reason for Paula's emergency caesarean section was a cord prolapse that necessitated a speedy delivery, and although a consent form for the operation was signed, it was very difficult to take everything in given the short time available. Hospital staff will usually take time after the delivery to talk to women, explaining what will happen and helping them make sense of their experience. However, Paula felt that in her case this did not happen, and she was left feeling confused and isolated:

I don't think they really understood how I felt. The general impression given was that I should pull myself together, and anyway I had a healthy baby and that was the only important thing. On reflection I suppose that made me feel guilty, of course having a healthy baby is important, but I need to talk through and grasp things for myself – nobody understood or tried to do this.

Paula did understand that the baby was healthy, but she was having difficulty in accepting her experience and still felt that the baby was not really hers. The only explanation Paula did receive did not help her perception of her experience:

On one occasion the doctors had been in to see me and I think there must have been students there, because he went into great detail about it all. Not for my benefit, he ignored me, but talked to the students. I really resented that, and then he went on to tell me how lucky I was, as though I should give him a medal, and wasn't I the failure. After he'd gone I cried buckets.

On Paula's discharge from hospital, she healed well physically but, looking back, felt that the first few weeks of Jessica's life were a blur. Paula was left unable to recall times, events and emotions. Paula's experience was compounded by her further contacts with health professionals. The community midwife seemed unaware of her problems, and Paula found the health visitor's attitude threatening.

Paula developed panic attacks and found it difficult to answer the front door. She also developed a fear of Jessica being taken away. Steve was aware that she was experiencing difficulties but was unsure what the best course of action was. Both sets of grandparents lived out of the region, and little family support was available. Some support came from close friends who were aware of Paula's experiences.

I don't feel that I got as much help as was possible, especially from the hospital. But at the time I was too immersed in it all to feel anything really. I just felt pretty numb, like I didn't register what was going on around me. A bit like being in a mental fog.

Paula got through her experiences with the support of Steve and a few close friends. Her experience with health professionals was such that she was reluctant to seek further help. Admitting to another health professional how she felt would almost have been like admitting to being a failure as a mother. Paula also expressed a fear of becoming addicted to medication. She also found it difficult to contact her parentcraft group for support:

I had a picture of the other women in my classes all going through labour well, breastfeeding and everything. Everything going well for them, how it should have gone for me. I thought that it was just me, unable to be a proper mother, that something was lacking in me. I was an unnatural woman, unable to do things properly.

Paula said of her experience that it had left her a totally changed person and that her relationship with Steve was also permanently changed. Paula was unable to state whether she had recovered from her experience as she still woke up with nightmares and sweats. The turning point probably came when Paula felt able to return to work part time:

I started to work part-time, regain my sense of self and worth. As Jessica grows I also know that I am her mother regardless and that I have redefined my definitions of motherhood.

Is it possible to relate Paula's experience of depression to the trauma of her birth experience? Other factors may have contributed to this situation. Paula herself identified that her expectations of motherhood were perhaps unrealistic and that neither herself nor Steve had any practical experiences of parenting. In addition, there was no family support available in the immediate vicinity. It would also appear that when she most needed support, Paula experienced a degree of isolation as she felt unable to contact the women that she had met during her pregnancy.

■ CASE HISTORY 2 ■

Psychological trauma

This was Susan's third pregnancy, her other children being 3 and 5 years old. Her two previous pregnancies and births were straightforward and uneventful. This was not a planned pregnancy, but both Susan and Gareth were pleased:

We had not consciously decided to have another baby but we hadn't ruled out any more children either. So when I found out I was pregnant again it was a surprise but I suppose I was quite pleased.

Having had two uneventful births, Susan decided that she would like to have this baby at home. This was discussed with Gareth, and they both decided that this was what they wanted:

A home birth seemed such a natural thing to do. Both my previous births had been relatively easy and so we couldn't see that there was any problem. We knew that there are very few home births these days but were still keen on the idea.

Susan made her first visit to her GP, who automatically suggested the local hospital. Susan then told the GP about her plans for this pregnancy:

He was very negative, horrified really and adamant that I was making a big mistake. There was no arguing. I was told that did I realise I was putting the life of my baby at risk. I went home feeling awful and really upset, booked for the local unit.

Susan was booked into the local hospital but was not happy with the way in which she was treated. She felt that she was not given a reasonable explanation of why a home birth was out of the question and why she was being treated as an irresponsible woman. Susan decided to shelve the idea of a home birth, and her pregnancy progressed normally. By chance, she discovered from a relative that she was entitled to give birth at home if she wanted to and that a local midwife would have to attend:

I felt really annoyed that I had been misinformed and that in fact I could have a home birth if that was what I wanted. So I went back to my GP and contacted the local hospital for my information.

Susan felt that she had come up against a brick wall. Home births were extremely unusual in the area where she lived. The GP spelt out graphically the dangers of postpartum haemorrhage and breathing problems with the baby and said that he would not be held responsible for any ensuing disaster.

The lack of support or balanced information was incredible, I really felt out on a limb. But that just made me more determined.

Susan's next encounter was with her community midwife manager and her community midwife, who made it plain that although they would provide two midwives to support her at her home birth, did she realise what a burden she was putting on the midwifery service? She was also instructed that she would need to ask her consultant's permission:

At 34 weeks pregnant I went back to the hospital to see my consultant who gave me a vivid account of a dreadful home birth he had witnessed years ago. He then turned to Gareth and said 'I would not allow my wife to behave so irresponsibly'. But basically I had got myself armed with information and knew there was nothing he could do about it.

Susan's confidence in her ability to give birth at home was constantly undermined by her community midwife's persistently negative comments. She felt that she was continually being pressurised to give in and go to the hospital, but her belief that she was making the right choice stayed firm.

A few days past her expected date of delivery, Susan went into labour and, as instructed, she contacted the community midwife, who came out to visit her and then went away again saying nothing was happening and to phone when things were more established. This was at 3 in the afternoon. By 3.30 p.m., Susan felt that she was contracting strongly and that she was definitely in good labour. Again, she contacted the midwife who was very negative down the phone.

What she told me was that I was fussing and that I should go into hospital for some pain relief. If I couldn't cope with niggling pains how did I think I would cope with proper labour at home. I insisted I was in labour and she said she would come out again. Almost like I was wasting her time.

When the midwife arrived, she seemed very put out by it all, and Susan felt that she was rough in the way she examined her. On examination, it was found that Susan was in the second stage of labour and the second midwife was called. The midwife remained uncommunicative and busied herself with her equipment until the second midwife arrived.

The midwife hardly spoke to me, but I didn't care by then. I don't even remember the second midwife arriving.

The midwives then told Susan that her labour was not progressing and she would have to go into hospital before the baby became distressed. However, Susan felt that everything was fine and that she would be unwise to move so late in labour. However, she was feeling increasingly undermined and emotionally distressed. Thomas was actually born at 5 p.m. and was in good condition. Had she taken the advice of the midwives he would have been born on the way to hospital.

All they could say was, how lucky I was that he was all right. I know he was all right. I think it was their lack of skills not a problem with my labour.

Over the next week, her relationship with her midwives continued to be poor, and she was having difficulty with establishing breastfeeding. Each midwife that visited gave out different information or presumed that, as this was her third baby, she would just get on with it. Thomas was slow to feed. Susan was not getting much sleep and kept focusing on the attitudes of the midwives during her pregnancy. By 3 weeks post-delivery, Gareth suggested that she went to the GP, who in turn was not very interested in Susan's distress. The couple decided that a change in GP would be a good idea and eventually found a new GP. By this time, Susan was having difficulty sleeping, was waking with nightmares and was finding everyday activities difficult. Susan's new GP felt that she was probably suffering from depression and recommended a course of medication along with input from the practice psychologist:

I had a good explanation of how the medication worked and having somebody who treated me with respect again made such a difference. The psychologist talked through everything with me which was so helpful.

Susan strongly believes that the conflicts and lack of support she experienced through her pregnancy were directly responsible for her emotional problems afterwards. Perhaps, in these circumstances, the last words should be left with Susan:

I had no problems with Lucy and Daniel so why should I have a problem this time? My big mistake was to not change GP earlier. I had

no confidence in the midwives but felt I was in a corner. Their attitude deprived me of what should have been a positive and happy
experience.

■ CASE HISTORY 3 ■

Reactivation of negative past experience

This was Lindsay's first pregnancy. Lindsay had not been in her
relationship long and the pregnancy was not planned. She had
only just finished her midwifery course; her partner was still a
student.

It came as a shock to find out I was pregnant, I hadn't got my number
through [registration as a qualified midwife] and I just wasn't ready for
this, at that point in my life. Mark was in his third year at college and
this was the year of his finals and getting a job. We were stunned.

Lindsay had an antepartum haemorrhage at 25 weeks pregnant and was admitted to hospital. A scan revealed that she had
a placenta praevia, which would necessitate an elective caesarean section and a reasonably long period of hospitalisation.

It was really weird because one minute I'm working in the hospital and
the next I'm a patient and it felt so strange.

Lindsay was kept in hospital for 8 weeks, was then allowed
home for a weekend and bled heavily. She was rushed to theatre
for an emergency caesarean section. Liam was born prematurely at 33 weeks and taken up to the neonatal unit.

Although I knew that this was a strong possibility, when it actually
happened it was a real shock and I was terrified.

Physically, Lindsay made a good recovery from her operation
and was happy with the treatment she received. What Lindsay
found difficult was having Liam on the neonatal unit, and Mark
found everything very difficult to cope with:

Mark found it all very stressful, he was having to work hard and then
coming in to visit. It was very hard for him and I'm sure he frequently
felt isolated.

Prior to starting her midwifery course, Lindsay had worked in a neonatal unit for some time, and so she was technically used to the neonatal intensive care environment. Also Liam was doing well.

First all those things I've heard people complain of again and again. They were all there, all of them. And when I had my roaring part at three days, I was weepy in the morning and then I got better in the afternoon, but being staff I just had a constant stream of visitors day and night. By the evening again I was really tired and got a bit weepy again. I'd been a bit weepy that morning when the night staff went off, and when the nurse came on that night I was weeping again. She said 'still crying are we?' and walked off.

Being a previous neonatal nurse and also a midwife had an effect on the way in which Lindsay was treated by the hospital staff. She was assumed to be competent at basic childcare skills. For Lindsay to admit that she was not confident felt like admitting defeat both as a professional and as a mother. No help was offered and so none was sought.

Liam did well on the neonatal unit, and after a few weeks both Lindsay and Liam were fit to return home. Liam was bottle-fed but Lindsay was not entirely comfortable with this:

I know I had awful guilt feelings about the fact that I wasn't breast-feeding as I thought I ought to be. Perhaps I didn't have the right kind of support at the beginning as well.

Lindsay planned to start work when Liam was 4 months old. Shortly prior to returning to work, she began to experience difficulties. Going out became a traumatic experience, and she was experiencing increasingly frequent episodes of crying:

It was just like, just suddenly I started to feel like this. And for a number of days then, I used to have the same kind of thing, uncontrollable crying, for no obvious reason.

Lindsay returned back to her job as a newly qualified midwife. The working environment she returned to had a fast pace, with poor staffing levels, and she was frequently left unsupported to cope alone:

I just started to worry terribly about work. I'm quite organised, good at managing lots of things at once. Then I found that I couldn't manage things like eat and talk at the same time, never mind juggle lots of things at work.

Lindsay had started to avoid friends; her social life, already affected by the pregnancy and birth of Liam, ground to a halt. Mark was wrapped up in his work. Everyday activities such as shopping became highly stressful:

Like, er, I was going to, the noise, the lights, the bustle. All the stuff around, it was like everything was going to fall in on top of me.

This hypersensitivity crossed over into different areas of Lindsay's life: worrying excessively about Liam, fanatical about harm coming to him and fearing that she would inadvertently become the source of that harm. Ideas of harm then became connected with self-harm:

It gradually turned into me. I wanted to kill myself. If this is my life I can't live it.

It was at this point when Lindsay was at her lowest, questioning her ability as a mother and her ability as a midwife, that she began experiencing nightmares relating to her experiences as a health professional:

Until that time I hadn't really thought enough about what it means when a baby dies. Having your own baby makes you think hard. How could I have worked with those babies and not been affected by them? In fact I was affected, it just came out then.

The nightmares of the sick and dying babies became intermingled during the day. Lindsay had now started to engage in arguments with Mark, whom she felt did not at that time have any idea of what she was suffering.

This situation developed over almost a year. Eventually, at one of Liam's developmental check-ups the health visitor observed something was wrong and got Lindsay a prompt appointment with the GP:

My GP is brilliant. I went into him, I couldn't speak, all of a sudden it was safe and I could speak, then I wept and wept.

With the combined help of her GP, health visitor and a community psychiatric nurse, Lindsay received medication and counselling. This support also included Mark, who had begun to realise that something was wrong but had no idea of the severity or how to handle it.

It took months before I knew what better was. It took months to realise that I would never be like I was before.

Part of Lindsay's counselling addressed the issue of the nightmares. Lindsay felt that, as a pregnant health professional, it was assumed that the skills of motherhood would come easily. What she actually found was that her experiences as a neonatal nurse, and to some extent as a midwife, had distorted her view of babies, leaving her mechanically skilled to cope with very sick babies but unable to deal psychologically with the demands of a healthy baby. Yet there was no support available to help her deal with her initial experiences as they occurred or to cope with her own first-hand experiences of motherhood.

Lindsay's postnatal depression may also have been affected by the fact that she was in a relationship where children were not yet part of the agenda. Her pregnancy was complicated by placenta praevia and a caesarean section culminating in the premature birth of Liam who went to the neonatal unit. All of this occurred at a time when Lindsay was not yet established in her working environment and Mark was embarking upon his important final year at college.

■ CASE HISTORY 4 ■

Inadequate social support networks

Sylvia married Craig at 20 and became pregnant almost immediately. At this stage in her life, Sylvia had no contact with her family, who lived several hundred miles away. Also, Sylvia had yet to forge a relationship with her new in-laws, having recently moved to be with her new husband.

The pregnancy was medically uncomplicated, but Sylvia found the birth of her daughter a long process.

I don't remember much about it as I'd had a couple of injections which made me woozy. Tracey was born and I just didn't want to look at her, I was so drugged, they wouldn't let me hold her. Craig wasn't allowed in the delivery room anyway. I'm glad he wasn't there, I didn't want him to see me in that state.

Sylvia had wanted to breast-feed Tracey as she had been breast-fed and felt it was the right thing to do, but at that time hospital policies dictated that babies were kept in the nursery and brought to mothers for 4-hourly feeding. Sylvia found that Tracey had already been given a bottle-feed.

When she were brought into me I couldn't feel anything for her. In the hospital the nurses ended up totally looking after her, I just refused to have anything to do like.

During the first few months of Tracey's life Sylvia coped alone with her new daughter:

It seemed like I was never going to ever have a night to myself again. There she was like a little changeling, as I saw her, and she was always demanding something. I used to hate it when she'd cry and I couldn't shut her up.

Sylvia also found that the night disturbances were her responsibility and that Craig did not like having his sleep disturbed:

I was really tired during the day and Craig used to moan if his supper weren't laid for him.

Occasionally, Sylvia's mother-in-law would call around, but the visits felt more critical than helpful:

When she came around it was to see our Tracey, not to help me. She usually visited when Craig was in so I'd end up brewing for the pair of them. I suppose it were her fault that he was that way, he'd always been waited on and it were right to him that I should do the same.

When Tracey was about 4 months old, Sylvia consulted her GP because she was worried about her own lack of sleep. During the day, Sylvia was exhausted, but she was unable to sleep at night as her mind was constantly racing.

I suppose Tracey was getting on for about 4 months when I began to get the voices. It sounds silly now, but at the time I was terrified!

Eventually, Sylvia was afraid to go to bed because that was when the voices started, so she would stay up doing housework, anything rather than going to bed. At this stage, Craig was working as a driver doing long hauls, so Sylvia was isolated at home.

So I took myself down the doctor's and said I hadn't slept proper since the babe had been born, and at first all he said was that babies were hard work and that it was unusual to sleep well in the first few months.

Having plucked up the courage to see her doctor only to be told that what she was feeling was normal was too much for Sylvia, who broke down in tears. Sylvia was given medication, which continued for about 6 years. Craig was annoyed that Sylvia had resorted to medication and found it to be another burden:

He wasn't pleased when he found out that I'd been to the doctors for the pills in the first place. He said that I shouldn't need to drug myself up, and that I only had the one baby, lots of people had far more to cope with than me.

In the 6 years that Sylvia was on medication, there was never any evaluation of the prescription: it was simply repeated. Sylvia became dependent upon the tablets, and it was on her own initiative that she managed to break with them:

It was very hard, but as I'd flushed them down the loo, I didn't have much choice.

Coming off the tablets left Sylvia shaky and panicky but she found that these feelings were not as bad as the feelings she had experienced after Tracey's birth. Eventually, Sylvia felt ready to do some part-time work. At first, working out of the house after over 6 years was a major hurdle, but the lunch-time bar work brought a new lease for Sylvia:

At first I thought that I would find it dead hard, but it was a relief to get out of the house. It was great just to get out and we used to have a good laugh and that.

On reflection, Sylvia felt that she had little experience of child-care and nobody to support her. She had moved away from close friends and family when she married Craig, and then became pregnant shortly afterwards, so there was no support available from her old home and she had not had time to establish new friends. Sylvia did not appear to have a good relationship with her mother-in-law. Craig was finding parenting difficult, working long hours to cope with the loss of Sylvia's earnings, and held the expectation that Sylvia should bring up Tracey whilst running the house as before. Sylvia's experience of Tracey's birth and her hospital stay was not positive. She had had a long labour and felt so heavily drugged that she was unable to relate to Tracey shortly after her birth. It is possible that had Sylvia had an adequate support network around her when Tracey was born, many of her negative experiences could have been avoided. Further to this, had Sylvia's GP monitored her use of the medication she was given, it is likely that she would not have taken it for 6 years. Sylvia would perhaps have benefited from counselling support, but this was never an option for her. Again, it is possible to highlight a combination of factors that can contribute to an individual's experience of postnatal depression.

■ CASE HISTORY 5 ■

Loss of self-identity

Jen was Kate and Ted's first baby. Kate married at 18 and Jen was born when Kate was 21. Up to this time Kate was working full time as an overlocker in the local textile industry.

Kate's experience of Jen's birth was generally positive, although it was 6 hours after the birth before Kate was able to see her daughter:

They said that she was born so quickly that they needed to give her a bit of oxygen, and just keep an eye on her and that's why I was left.

Kate chose to bottle-feed Jen and felt that the hospital routine of 4-hourly feeds meant that she got a good rest whilst she was in hospital:

They used to take the babies out, feed them and bring them back once they'd fed. We had a sister who was brilliant, who thought that not just babies needed the rest, mums did as well.

Initially, Kate had her mother and Ted with her. Problems started to occur 2 weeks after Jen's birth when Ted returned to work and her mum returned to her own home. Kate found that suddenly to be on her own was 'horrible'. It seemed to Kate that there were just not enough hours in the day:

I remember one particular night, Ted didn't get home till about half five. I'd started his dinner. Jen had woken up and she wanted feeding. He walked in and he said there was something burning. I'd burnt the dinner. I went berserk. Little things like that could set me off. I just didn't want to go out. I wouldn't bother with myself.

Kate felt that if friends came around they were no longer coming around to see her, it was just the baby they wanted to see. Kate was also very aware that of all their friends, Ted and herself were the first couple to have children.

Before if we wanted to go out, we'd go. I think that this is a big thing that stops. At the least stupid thing I felt inadequate.

These feelings of inadequacy increased and with increased inadequacy came loss of sleep as Kate desperately struggled to plan her day in advance. She felt she could not relax and was desperately trying to cope with her new role as a mother.

It's lovely when you have your baby, but how can I put it? What people say and that, can adjust the scales that little bit.

Kate found that the loss of independence she had experienced was very difficult to come to terms with and that it was hard to try and blend the strands of her life.

Mind you I had a good GP in them days. He said that it was a natural thing what I was feeling and I could just sit and talk to him.

Kate however found that, although on a practical level her mother was a great help, she did not understand Kate's feelings:

I'm the eldest of four. I just don't think she could understand why I was like it.

Ted noticed that Kate was not her usual self and contacted her sister Jo to see whether she could help. Jo took Kate away, Jen now being 12 months old, cared for her and then just listened:

I felt much better, there again because she wasn't telling me what I had to do. She was just sitting there listening.

Kate found she'd be better for a short while and then slide back into depressions.

Now I think you have to get your priorities right. Half the problem was if I think about it, overtiredness. You just knacker yourself up.

On top of this Kate identified how difficult it was to make the change from work to home:

A lot is boredom, lack of company, feed, change, then out in the pram. Jen were born in November, so it was winter. You didn't go too far, it was either bitterly cold, or snowing. You were like penned in four walls till husband came home.

As all Kate's friends were childless and still working full time, she lost contact with many of them, and this accentuated her isolation and perhaps also the loss of her former identity. Kate's recovery was a gradual process of progress and slight regression. When Jen was 2 years old, Kate found her a nursery place and returned to work part time. However, Kate found this unsatisfactory as she felt she was missing out on Jen's development, so she left work only to return when Jen was well established at school. Kate found herself in a situation in which she was the first of her peer group to become a mother. All her friends were in full-time employment, which essentially left Kate isolated not only from her peer group, but also from her former lifestyle. No longer free to socialise readily at night and isolated from peer group socialising during the day, she faced a possible loss of identify. Kate's old identity was replaced with the identity of full-time mother, which she found very demanding and difficult to organise. Kate, having been competent in her work and lifestyle, suddenly found that she was unable to cope with the demands of a small baby, making her feel inadequate and incompetent. The situation was possibly aggravated by the attitude of her mother, who had brought up four children and was apparently unable to understand how Kate felt.

Conclusion

This chapter has been concerned with the classification of postnatal depression as a psychiatric disorder. The advantages and disadvantages of such a classification have been clearly identified. Five case

126

histories were presented to illustrate the range of factors associated with the onset of postnatal depression and maternal distress. The complexity of the women's experiences should not be underestimated, but a commonly recurring theme would appear to be a sense of loss of control and ensuing feelings of helplessness. In all of the case histories presented, the women experienced postnatal depression following pregnancies that were, at least initially, presumed to be normal, and although the experiences of birth varied in terms of the levels of trauma involved, the women all gave birth to live, healthy babies. Nevertheless, the levels of distress and pain involved were considerable. The next chapter considers maternal distress in instances where things have clearly gone badly for the women involved.

References

Brown, G. W. and Harris, T. O. (1978) *The Social Origins of Depression* (London: Tavistock).

Cox, J. and Holden, J. (eds) *Perinatal Psychiatry, Use and Misuse of Edinburgh Postnatal Depression Scale* (London: Gaskell).

Doyal, L. (1995) *What makes Women Sick?* (London: Macmillan).

DSM IV (1995) Diagnostic and Statistical Manual of Mental Disorders (Washington DC: American Psychiatric Association).

Elliott, S., Sanjack, M. and Leverton, J. J. (1988) 'Parent Groups in Pregnancy: a preventative intervention for postnatal depression?' In Gottlieb, B. H. (ed.) *Marshalling Social Support* (London: Sage Publications).

Gilbert, P. (1992) *Depression: The Evolution of Powerlessness* (Hove: Lawrence Erlbaum).

Kitzinger, S. (1992) 'Birth and Violence Against Women: Generating Hypotheses from Women's Accounts of Unhappiness after Childbirth.' In Roberts, H. (ed.) *Women's Health Matters* (London: Routledge).

Oakley, A. (1993) *Essays on Women, Medicine and Health* (Edinburgh: Edinburgh University Press).

O'Hara, M. W., Zekoski, E. M., Phillips, Z. H. and Wright, E. J. (1990) 'A Controlled Prospective Study of Post Partum Mood Disorders: Comparison of Childbearing and Non-childbearing women.' *Journal of Abnormal Psychology* **99**: 3–15.

Rubel, A. J. (1979) 'Epidemiology of a Folk Illness: Susto in Hispanic America.' In Landy, D. (ed.) *Culture, Disease and Healing* (New York: Macmillan).

Russo, N. F. (1986) *Women's Mental Health Agenda* (Washington DC: American Psychological Association).

Showalter, E. (1987) *The Female Malady: Women, Madness and English Culture 1830–1979* (London: Virago).

Ussher, J. M. (1991) *Women's Madness: Misogyny or Mental Illness?* (Hemel Hempstead: Harvester/Wheatsheaf).

World Health Organization (1992) *International Classification of Diseases 10 (ICD 10)* (Geneva: WHO).

World Health Organization (1993) *Psychosocial and Mental Health Aspects of Women's Health* (Geneva: WHO).

Chapter 7

Motherhood, Loss and Distress Following Childbirth

This dissonance between personal knowing and expert knowing seemed to reinforce for the women that there were no guarantees, no way to make and keep everything right again, the way it was supposed to be.

(Marck et al., 1994, p. 280)

This chapter is concerned with loss and distress following childbirth. The first part of the chapter looks at the distressing factors associated with giving birth to a preterm baby. Maternal experiences of disempowerment and separation of the mother and baby will be discussed here. The second part of the chapter considers the additional stress factors associated with twins and multiple births. The third part of the chapter is concerned with maternal responses to giving birth to a mentally and/or physically impaired baby, whilst the fourth part deals with the long-term distress and disruption that may follow relinquishing a baby for fostering or adoption. Part five of the chapter looks at the multiple losses faced by mothers who are HIV-positive or are suffering from the acquired immune deficiency syndrome (AIDS), and the final part of the chapter introduces a general model of coping when motherhood is 'uncertain' (Field and Marck, 1994).

Preterm birth

Every year, between 40 000 and 50 000 babies will be born prematurely. Whilst the majority of these babies will survive, many will need to be nursed in a special care baby unit (SCBU). Babies who need intensive care will be placed on a neonatal unit (NNU). Preterm labour may be very sudden in origin, and such births are often characterised by high levels of medical intervention. Table 7.1 highlights some of the possible causes of preterm birth. However, in approximately 50 per cent of instances, the cause of preterm birth is unknown. The type of delivery will depend on the severity of cause, the period of gestation and professional assessments of the wellbeing (or otherwise) of the baby.

Table 7.1   Causes of preterm birth

Cause	Some common symptoms
Abnormally shaped uterus	May cause labour to start early Uterine shape may be detected by scan or fetal presentation
Antepartum haemorrhage (APH)	Bleeding from genital tract Abdominal tenderness Signs of maternal shock if severe
Chronic maternal illness	Dependent upon type of illness
Congenital abnormality	Associated with elevated risk of preterm birth
Incompetent cervix	Associated with elevated risk of preterm birth
Irritable uterus	Early experience of intermittent uterine contractions, which in some cases develops into labour
Maternal infection	Raised white blood cell count, pyrexia, irritable uterus, general malaise Ultimately dependent upon source and type of infection
Multiple pregnancy	Associated with elevated risk of preterm birth
Polyhydramnios	Uterus palpates larger than expected size for dates
Pre-eclampsia	Headaches, oedema, oliguria, raised blood pressure, epigastric pain, visual disturbances, epileptic-type seizures
Pregnancy-induced hypertension (PIH)	Raised maternal blood pressure Impaired renal function Possible growth retardation of the fetus
Renal disease (pyelonephritis)	Raised maternal blood pressure Poor fetal growth Urinary complications
Spontaneous rupture of the membranes (SROM)	Leakage of amniotic fluid – can be confused with urinary incontinence
Stress and emotional factors	Associated with elevated risk of preterm birth

Adapted from Sweet (1988).

In certain cases, the cause of preterm birth will be unknown. Furthermore, relatively few women will have any amount of time in which to anticipate the fact that they will give birth prematurely. Babies who are born preterm have a high risk of dying and suffering from a physical and/or mental impairment compared with babies who are born at full term. Consequently, maternal anxiety is characteristically high. Taylor and Littlewood (1993) considered preterm birth passages to be so atypical from normal deliveries that they developed a different model of the 'passage' from one state to another in the instance of preterm birth. This alternative model is given in Table 7.2.

Table 7.2 Preterm birth as an abnormal transition

Passage	Preterm maternal experiences
I Separation (mother and child)	Unlike full-term birth, preterm birth occurs at no particular time Often considered to be an emergency rather than a 'normal' sequence of events
2 Transition (labour)	Increased shock and anxiety No planning for labour Unsafe delivery The baby may be taken away
3 Re-incorporation (from hospital to community)	Experience on postnatal ward may be absent or upsetting Mother may go home without the baby No celebrations because of concern about condition of the baby

Adapted from Taylor (1992).

Given a traumatic delivery and concern over the future health of her baby, the most characteristic feelings associated with mothers of preterm babies are shock, disorientation and acute anxiety. Any taken-for-granted understanding of the process of pregnancy and childbirth the woman may have had is likely to be severely violated by her actual experience.

If the baby is admitted to an NNU, anxiety may be compounded by loss. The 'ideal' baby the woman may have expected to have is lost (Sherr, 1989) and the anticipated role of primary caregiver has also been lost. (Kennell *et al.*, 1970). Furthermore, the specialist and highly technical nature of the care given on NNUs has been shown to make mothers feel both incompetent and superfluous in terms of their perception of their abilities to care for their babies (Gottlieb, 1978).

As Stainton (1985) indicates, contact with and caring for the baby facilitates a sense of the maternal competence, as does the baby's responsiveness to care giving. When a baby is born preterm and hospitalised on a NNU, the mothering role is difficult to realise, so maternal activities that focus on 'getting to know' the baby are severely inhibited.

Brady-Fryer (1994) looked at multiparous women who experienced a preterm birth and identified the following sources of distress:

- Preterm birth;
- The initial appearance of the baby;
- Shock at the high levels of technology used to support the infant;
- Feelings of disempowerment;
- Difficulties in relating to NNU staff;
- Discharge from hospital.

The mothers in Brady-Fryer's study sought a cause for giving birth preterm. The overwhelming feeling following preterm birth was frequently one of failure. The initial appearance of the baby also gave mothers cause for concern.

The NNU itself may be found to be intimidating and shocking. The high levels of technology required to support some babies, coupled with the high levels of expertise required to manipulate it, left many mothers feeling disempowered:

It's such a feeling of helplessness and frustration, of futility and useless-ness, standing there and being no earthly use to your own baby.

(Brady-Fryer, 1994, p. 203)

In such a situation, expressing breast milk to feed their babies was shown to minimise the mothers' sense of frustration (Brady-Fryer, 1994; Taylor and Littlewood, 1994).

Many mothers experienced difficulties in relating to hospital staff following preterm birth (Brady-Fryer, 1994; Taylor, 1992). Further-more, the discharge of the mother, in some instances without her baby, was also experienced as a source of anxiety and distress.

Whilst Brady-Fryer (1994) indicates that mothers of preterm infants eventually 'forged a role' for themselves and went on success-fully to care for their baby, she also indicates that whilst maternal feelings of guilt and disappointment receded, a sense of loss and sadness remained. However, 'forging a role' was dependent upon mothers receiving consistent social support in their efforts to mother their preterm babies.

Taylor and Littlewood (1994) and Littlewood and Taylor (1996) found that, in instances where mothers were given conflicting advice, the mothers in their sample expressed high levels of anxiety and distress. Furthermore, maternal concern over the long-term development of the child was also present in the women they interviewed.

Twins and multiple births

The pregnancy, delivery and care of twins and multiple births have been shown to be more stressful compared with the mothers of singletons. The greater psychological conflict amongst mothers expecting a multiple birth has also been documented (Thorpe *et al.*, 1991). In addition to the feelings of ambivalence common to most mothers upon confirmation of their pregnancy, conflicts relating to the extra financial and health burdens of bearing twins have been identified (see, for example, Spillman, 1984, 1987). In spite of feelings of pride about being exceptional, ambivalence, shock, depression and anger upon learning of a multiple pregnancy have been found to be almost universal (Scheinfield, 1973).

For the mothers of twins, the pregnancy may be more physically and emotionally stressful compared with that of mothers of singletons. Bodily discomfort may be exacerbated, with feelings of heaviness occurring at an earlier stage in the pregnancy. The mothers of multiple births also experience an increased risk of obstetric problems. For example, preterm labour, fetal growth retardation and pre-eclampsia have all been associated with multiple births (Linney, 1983). As a consequence, mothers are more frequently monitored and obstetric interventions are more likely. Obviously, in such a situation maternal anxiety is likely to be increased. Unfortunately, the outcome of multiple births in terms of special care, congenital abnormalities and perinatal mortality is poorer compared with that of single births (Magnus *et al.*, 1990).

In the months following the birth, difficulties in coping with sleeping patterns, which are often unsynchronised, and with feeding and crying patterns may lead to additional fatigue and exhaustion. Furthermore, the logistics of taking two or more infants out at the same time may lead to the mother simply staying at home and, as a result, experiencing isolation (Haigh and Wilkinson, 1989).

Feelings of guilt concerning the ability, or lack of it, to give adequate and equal attention to more than one baby have also been frequently reported in the literature (see, for example, Robin et al., 1988). Such feelings may be greater for mothers who have other children who require attention. In such circumstances, it should not surprise us to note that the incidence of child abuse is greater in families of twins (Nelson and Martin, 1985).

The available evidence would suggest that the additional stress associated with giving birth to more than one baby at the same time may be long term. For example, Powell (1981) conducted a study of first-born twins and found that, in the first year of motherhood, mothers of twins reported more symptoms of stress (particularly anxiety and fatigue) than did matched control singleton mothers. Furthermore, Haigh and Wilkinson (1989) noted a disturbing trend in which the proportion of mothers with twins experiencing depression and anxiety tended to increase over time whilst that of a control group of singleton mothers decreased.

Clearly, whilst twins and multiple births are often associated with feelings of pride and achievement, the available evidence indicates that they are also associated with an increased risk of maternal distress and depression.

Giving birth to a mentally and/or physically impaired baby

Maternal responses to giving birth to a mentally and/or physically impaired baby have been likened to grief by some researchers in the area (see, for example, Irvin et al., 1982). As with preterm birth, the 'distance' between the woman's 'ideal fantasy baby' and her real baby may indeed be great (Solnit and Stark, 1961). It may take some time before a mother comes to love her impaired baby (Roberts, 1977). Similar to experiences of bereavement, uncertainty over who the baby actually is and what is being mourned may be felt by the mother of an impaired baby (Mander, 1994).

Another significant feature of maternal response to the birth of an impaired baby is occasional feelings that the child might be better off dead (Lewis and Bourne, 1989). Many women find these thoughts to be alarming, and Mander (1994) suggests that they may both aggravate guilt and trigger depression. Roberts (1977) suggests that warning mothers of impaired babies of the possibility of such thoughts occurring may help to allay their concerns.

However, Leon (1990) suggests that the birth of an impaired baby represents a major narcissistic injury to the woman's self-esteem. This feeling may be aggravated by the presence of an impaired child, which serves to remind the woman of the loss of her 'fantasy' baby and of her own sense of failure (Raphael-Leff, 1991). Raphael (1984) makes a similar point and suggests that each 'developmental milestone' so easily reached by non-impaired babies may serve to retrigger the sense of loss in mothers who have given birth to an impaired baby.

These experiences may unfortunately be compounded in some instances by the relatively higher risks of premature mortality associated with some impairments. Paradoxically, the woman's very adjustment to her impaired child can, in certain instances, sharpen the feelings of loss and complicate grief following the death of an impaired baby. For example, a woman whose much-loved youngest daughter had Down's syndrome, and eventually died from leukaemia, expressed intense sorrow and perceptions of unfairness regarding her daughter's death. Other people's perception of the death as 'a blessing' did much to fuel her anger (at others, and at herself because she had occasionally had similar thoughts herself) and did nothing to assuage her grief.

Diachuk (1994) looked specifically at maternal adjustment to the birth of a baby with Down's syndrome in women who already had other children. Her study took place whilst the children were relatively young, and she charted the gradual process of acceptance in the mothers she studied in the following way:

When they were informed of the diagnosis of Down Syndrome there was initial denial, followed by maternal acceptance. At first the mothers were uncertain about their own ability to care for their new-borns, but they soon began to focus upon the normality of the babies rather than on the diagnosis. They had a need to be able to take control in order to assume the role of mother. This increased their perceptions of maternal competence. Another critical factor was the acceptance of the children as members of both the immediate and extended family and of the wider community.

(Diachuk, 1994, p. 266)

However, it must be said that deviance from Diachuk's model could occur at any point within it, and the impact of poor professional help and failure of communal support is not illuminated by her work.

Relinquishing a baby for fostering or adoption

As Morris (1983) has indicated, it used to be thought that relinquishing a baby for fostering or adoption at the time of birth was unrelated to any sense of loss because;

> adoption is a voluntary act on the woman's behalf [so] it somehow appears different. And the need to mourn for her child may therefore go unrecognised by those who care for her.
>
> *(Morris, 1983, p. 33)*

Alternatively Rolls *et al.* (1986) and Sorosky *et al.* (1984) argue strongly that grieving following adoption has many features in common with loss by death. However, Mander (1994) quite rightly points out that there are certain crucial differences between relinquishing a child for adoption and experiencing the death of a child. In particular, Mander argues that 'grief' following relinquishment is frequently complicated because of the common circumstances surrounding relinquishment. Firstly, Mander questions the 'voluntary' nature of relinquishing and points out that many women relinquish for external rather than internal reasons. Furthermore, these external social reasons also tend to involve pressurising the woman into secrecy about the relinquishment. The woman may be encouraged to get on with her life as if 'nothing had happened' and may find that her grief is reactivated at a later date, when she is less busy or in connection with some subsequent loss.

Littlewood (1992) and Cline (1995) have suggested that, even in normal grieving, people rarely 'let go' of their loss and that 'consolidation' is a better descriptive term for the latter parts of the process of grief. Mander takes this observation further in connection with the relinquishing mother and questions whether a woman who relinquishes her child can ever really comes to terms with her experience because of the very real hope, or fear, of contact with her child at some later date. This factor may impede grieving and leave a woman to feel that relinquishment can never really be concluded in any meaningful way.

Whilst people caring for a woman who has suffered the death of her newborn child have increasingly recognised her need to actively grieve for her loss, relinquishment, possibly due to perceptions concerning the 'voluntary' nature of the act, has only recently been associated with maternal distress. Furthermore, relinquishment may be an often hidden factor that has far-reaching consequences for the woman's life. For example, the following account of maternal distress and subsequent depression was volunteered to us at the beginning of our research for this book. Ms A wrote a letter in which she clearly documented her experiences 20 years previously.

■ CASE HISTORY 6 ■

Consequences of 'voluntary' relinquishment

Ms A was raped by a friend of her family and became pregnant at 16. Her family effectively disowned her and she was coerced into relinquishing her baby for adoption. Ms A felt that the atti-tude of the hospital staff was punitive. She recalled being told that she was a disgrace to her family, and the nursing staff refused to disclose the sex of her baby.

Upon being discharged from hospital, she received help from the Church and within 2 years found employment and married. She became pregnant with a second child, which she was deter-mined to bear. However, her partner failed to understand her desperate desire to bear a child and deserted her during her pregnancy. Following an uncomplicated labour, she gave birth to a healthy baby and tried to cope alone. She experienced flash-backs to her first traumatic labour and became convinced that her health visitor would take her baby away. Consequently, she refused to let her health visitor visit and became agoraphobic. Unfortunately, the history of Ms A's experiences were unknown to her health visitor and Ms A's worst fears were eventually realised when she was detained for inpatient treatment. Her baby was taken from her, and it took 16 years, together with the intervention of MIND, for Ms A to be released. Ms A never saw either of her children again. According to her letter, she thinks of them constantly and wrote to us in the hope that her appalling experiences could be useful in terms of preventing of any similar occurrences.

In connection with an earlier piece of work, Littlewood (1992) interviewed 'Mrs G'.

■ CASE HISTORY 7 ■
A multiple loss situation

Mrs G effectively suffered a triple loss involving an impaired baby, relinquishment by fostering and the death of her child. Mrs G's son had Down's syndrome and, as a single parent with two older children, Mrs G was pressurised by her family to opt for long-term fostering. Mrs G reluctantly agreed to this but subsequently doubted her decision. The couple who were fostering Mrs G's son had themselves lost a son who had Down's syndrome some years earlier. Unfortunately, this couple's affluence contrasted sharply with Mrs G's poverty, and although Mrs G longed for her son's return, she felt unable to ask for it due to her idea that he would be 'better off' with his foster parents. Nevertheless, Mrs G constantly fantasised about a time when she 'got everything sorted out' and her son would be returned to her. Mrs G's son died at his foster parents' home when he was 2 years old. Two years following the death, and after several psychiatric inpatient admissions, Mrs G remained inconsolable and ridden with guilt. Her anguish was compounded by her belief that she was a 'bad mother' who had no right to grieve for her son because 'it was me who rejected him and it was all my own fault for giving him away in the first place'.

Whilst all the losses dealt with in this chapter have the unfortunate tendency to multiply, it would appear that not all of them carry the potential for resolution.

Pregnancy and childbirth for women who are HIV-positive

Current knowledge of HIV/AIDS would indicate that those infected by the virus will experience a shortened life expectancy (Sherr, 1989). Furthermore, multiple losses may be said to characterise the lives of people affected. Whilst it is known that the prognosis for women is poorer than for men (Kell and Barton, 1991) the reasons for this remain unclear. However, there is no doubt that the losses associated with HIV/AIDS are extensive. Sherr (1989, 1991) identifies the following losses:

● Loss of life;

- Loss of health;
- Loss of relationships by avoidance, stigma and death;
- Loss of children, actual (by death or voluntary termination) or potential (by childlessness);
- Loss of self-image;
- Economic losses;
- Anticipation of and subsequent fear of losses;
- Loss of control due to illness and dependency upon others.

Obviously, an infection that may be transmitted by unprotected sexual intercourse should be a major cause for concern amongst women who want to bear children. However, characteristically enough, when concern over HIV/AIDS has been expressed in connection with pregnant women, that concern has been focused on the baby rather than the mother (Mander, 1994).

Pregnancy is a difficult issue for women who know of their HIV-positive status. A woman may desperately want a child if she knows that her lifespan will be relatively short. Alternatively, she may contemplate childlessness when she had previously assumed that she would have the option of having children at some later date.

Pregnancy was once thought to accelerate the progression of HIV through to AIDS (Lapointe *et al.*, 1984), and women with HIV who wish to become pregnant may be concerned over the impact that the pregnancy may have upon their health status. Alternatively, although questionably, rates of vertical transmission of the virus, that is, from mother to baby, have often been reported as being high (see, for example, the European Collaborative Study, 1991). Consequently, the mother may fear that she will jeopardise the health status of her baby. In addition, she may fear that she will damage the health of her baby in other ways (see, for example, Johnstone *et al.*, 1988).

Furthermore, a woman who discovers her HIV-positive status during a pregnancy will face previously unanticipated decisions concerning whether or not to continue with her pregnancy. For women who have existing, possibly uninfected, older children, exactly when and how to tell these children may cause anguish and guilt (Barlow, 1992). Fear of dying before her children gain independence and the associated loss for the mother of failing to observe the development of her children may also cause anguish and grief. Paradoxically, it may be the potentially overwhelming nature of these multiple losses that has led to the paucity of documented research concerning the support of women who are HIV-positive or have AIDS. Alternatively, the 'myth of Madonna' may have rendered an association between HIV-positive status/AIDS and maternity unthinkable for those who are not directly affected by the relevant issues. Nevertheless, research is urgently required in this area if we are to be able effectively to help women who are faced with such a daunting range of losses.

Unfortunately, the desire for pregnancy frequently and necessarily overcomes the practice of safer sex. Unless male fidelity can be assured, conception cannot be combined with HIV prevention. In societies in which motherhood represents the only route to status and identity, the position is particularly bleak. As one of de Bruyn's Ugandan respondents indicated:

> I don't mind dying but to die without a child means that I will have perished without trace. God will have cheated me.
>
> *(de Bruyn, 1992, p. 255)*

Marck *et al.*'s model of uncertain motherhood

Marck *et al.* (1994) have considered a range of losses associated with maternity and have offered a generic model of how women live through mothering experiences when the outcome is uncertain. This model is given in Figure 7.1.

Marck *et al.* suggest that women do not necessarily appraise and identify threats in the same way as do health professionals. For example, a woman embarking on a pregnancy following a stillbirth might appraise the threat of another stillbirth as being high, whilst a health professional may appraise it as being low. Furthermore, women tended to reduce the sense of threat to their images of motherhood by comparing themselves with other women in an attempt to 'normalise' their experiences. This would indicate that the presence of women who have undergone, or are undergoing, a similar experience should prove helpful.

Whilst self-protection could take a variety of forms depending upon the individual woman, all of the women considered by Marck *et al.* made efforts to protect themselves from loss or potential loss. Affect of control was achieved by the following combinations:

- Blaming oneself or others for the experience;
- 'Connecting', in order further to process and understand;
- 'Disconnecting', in order to 'buy time' to cope with the situation.

140

Figure 7.1 A general model of coping when the outcome of motherhood is uncertain

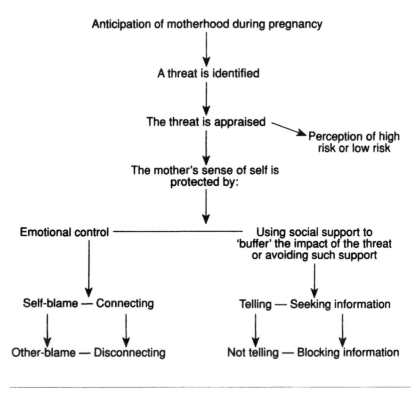

Anticipation of motherhood during pregnancy

A threat is identified

The threat is appraised → Perception of high risk or low risk

The mother's sense of self is protected by:

Emotional control ———————— Using social support to 'buffer' the impact of the threat or avoiding such support

Self-blame — Connecting   Telling — Seeking information

Other-blame — Disconnecting   Not telling — Blocking information

Adapted from Marck et al. *(1994).*

Clearly, women actively strive for an understanding of why a loss-related event happened in order to control the impact of the event upon them and/or to avoid the recurrence of a similar event. 'Stress buffering', either by seeking information and/or by social support, was also an activity used to cope with situations of loss and distress associated with maternity.

Conclusion

This chapter has considered a range of issues that are associated with loss and distress following childbirth. All of these issues are associated with long-term problems for the women who have to confront them. The losses involved were frequently multiple and some of the ways in which women attempted to cope with their loss have been discussed. The importance of appropriate and sensitive social support for mothers who face these distressing situations cannot be overemphasised. Nevertheless, the impact of the events described in this chapter is likely to be considerable, and any woman exposed to them will be permanently changed by her encounter. These changes will profoundly affect her orientation to any subsequent pregnancy upon which she embarks. However, in many ways the maternal distress addressed in this chapter is of a highly visible nature because something has very clearly 'gone wrong' with the outcome of the pregnancy. Consequently, subsequent maternal distress is not difficult either to understand or identify. Unfortunately, the distress associated with a baby dying at, or around the time of, birth is equally transparent. This will be the subject of Chapter 8.

References

Barlow, J. (1992) 'Social Issues: An Overview.' In Bury, J., Morrison, V. and Malachlan, S. (eds) *Working with Women and AIDS: Medical, Social and Counselling Issues* (London: Tavistock/Routledge).

Brady-Fyer, B. (1994) 'Becoming a Mother of a Pre-term Baby.' In Field, P. A. and Marck, P. B. (eds) *Uncertain Motherhood: Negotiating the Risks of the Childbearing Years* (London: Sage Publications).

Bruyn, M. de (1992) 'Women and AIDS in Developing Countries.' *Social Science and Medicine* **34**(3): 249–62.

Cline, S. (1995) *Lifting the Taboo: Women, Death and Dying* (London: Little, Brown and Company).

Diachuk, G. (1994) 'When a Child has a Birth Defect.' In Field, P. A. and Marck, P. B. (eds) *Uncertain Motherhood: Negotiating the Risks of the Childbearing Years* (London: Sage).

European Collaborative Study (1991) 'Children Born to Women with HIV Infection: Natural History and Risk of Transmission.' *Lancet* **337**(8736): 253–60.

Field, P. A. and Marck, P. B. (1994) *Uncertain Motherhood: Negotiating the Risks of the Child Bearing Years* (London: Sage Publications).

Gottlieb, L. 'Maternal Attachment in Primiparas.' *Journal of Obstetric, Gynecological and Neonatal Nursing* **7**(1): 39–44.

Haigh, J. and Wilkinson, L. (1989) 'Care and Management of Twins.' *Health Visitor* **62**: 43–5.

Irvin, N. A., Kennell, J. H. and Klaus, M. H. (1982) 'Caring for the Parents of an Infant with a Congenital Malformation.' In Klaus, M. and Kennell, J. (eds) *Parent–Infant Bonding*, 2nd edn (St Louis: C. V. Mosby).

Johnstone, F. D., MacCallum, L., Brettle, R., Inglis, J. M. and Peutherer, J. F. (1988) 'Does Infection with HIV Affect the Outcome of Pregnancy.' *British Medical Journal* **296**: 467.

Kell, P. and Barton. S. 'How do Women with HIV Present?' *Maternal and Child Health* **16**(11): 340–4.

Kennell, J., Slyter, H. and Klaus, M. M. (1970) 'The Mourning Responses of Parents on the Death of a Newborn Infant.' *New England Journal of Medicine* **283**: 344–9.

Lapointe, M., Michaud, J. and Pekovich, D. (1984) 'Transplacental Transmission of HTLV III Virus.' *New England Journal of Medicine* **312**: 1325–6.

Leon, I. G. (1990) *When a Baby Dies: Psychotherapy for Pregnancy and Newborn Loss* (Yale: Yale University Press).

Lewis, E. and Bourne, S. (1989) 'Perinatal Death.' In Oates, M. (ed.) *Psychological Aspects of Obstetrics and Gynaecology* (London: Baillière Tindall).

Linney, J. (1983) *Multiple Births* (London: Routledge and Kegan Paul).

Littlewood, J. (1992) *Aspects of Grief: Bereavement in Adult Life* (London: Routledge).

Littlewood, J. and Taylor, L. S. (1994) Postnatal care following premature birth, *Health Visitor* **67**(7): 235–7.

Littlewood, J. and Taylor, L. (1996) *The Breastfeeding Experiences of Mothers of Pre-term and Full-Term Infants.* Paper presented to 16th Annual Conference of the Society for Reproductive and Infant Psychology, Goldsmiths' College, University of London, September.

Magnus, P., Arntzen, A., Samuelson, S. O., Halderson, T. and Bakketeig, T. (1990) *No Correlation in Post-neonatal Deaths for Twins. A Study of the Early Mortality of Twins Based on the Norwegian Medical Birth Registry. Early Human Development* **223**: 89–97.

Mander, R. (1994) *Loss and Bereavement in Childbearing* (London: Blackwell Scientific).

Marck, P. B., Field, P. A. and Bergum, V. (1994) 'A Search for Understanding.' In Field, P. A. and Marck P. B. (eds) *Uncertain Motherhood: Negotiating the Risks of the Childbearing Years* (London: Sage Publications).

Morris, H. (1983) 'As Great a Loss.' *Nursing Mirror* February **16**: 33.

Nelson, M. H. B. and Martin, C. A. (1985) 'Increased Child Abuse in Twins.' *Child Abuse and Neglect* **9**: 502–5.

Powell, T. J. (1981) Symptoms of Postnatal (Atypical) Depression in Mothers of Twins. MSc thesis, University of Surrey.

Raphael, B. (1984) *The Anatomy of Bereavement: A Handbook for the Caring Professions* (London: Unwin Hyman)

Raphael-Leff, J. (1991) *Psychological Process of Childbearing* (London: Chapman & Hall).

Roberts, F. B. (1977) *Perinatal Nursing: Care of Newborns and their Families* (New York: McGraw-Hill).

Robin, M., Josse, D. and Tourette, C. (1988) 'Mother–Twin Interaction During Early Childhood.' *Acta Genetica Medica Gemelloia (Roma)* **37**: 151–9.

Rolls, S., Millen, L. and Backlund, B. (1986) 'Solomon's Mothers: Mourning in Mothers who Relinquish their Children for Adoption.' In Rando, T. A. (ed.) *Parental Loss of a Child* (Champaign: Illinois Research Press).

Scheinfield, A. (1973) *Twins and Supertwins* (Harmondworth: Penguin).

Sherr, L. (1989) *HIV and AIDS in Mothers and Babies* (Oxford: Blackwell Scientific).

Sherr, L. (ed.) (1989) *Death, Dying and Bereavement* (Oxford: Blackwell Scientific).

Solnit, A. J. and Stark, M. H. (1961) 'Mourning and the Birth of a Defective Child.' *Psychoanalytical Study of the Child* **16**: 523–37.

Sorosky, A. D., Baran, A. and Pannor, R. (1984) *The Adoption Triangle* (New York: Anchor).

Spillman, J. R. (1984) 'Double Exposure – Coping with Newborn Twins at Home.' *Midwife, Health Visitor and Community Nurse* **20**: 92.

Spillman, J. R. (1987) 'Emotional Aspects of Experiencing a Multiple Birth.' *Midwife, Health Visitor and Community Nurse* **23**: 54.

Stainton, C. M. (1985) Origins of Attachment: Culture and Cue Sensitivity Unpublished Doctoral Dissertation, University of California.

Sweet, B. R. (1988) *Mayes' Midwifery: A Textbook for Midwives*, 11th edn (London: Baillière Tindall).

Taylor, L. (1992) A Comparison of Maternal Experiences of Pre-term vs Full-Term Birth. Unpublished MA thesis, Loughborough University.

Taylor, L. S. and Littlewood, J. (1993) 'Premature Birth: Its Effects on Mothers.' *New Generations Digest* **2**: 10.

Taylor, L. S. and Littlewood, J. (1994) *The Breastfeeding Experiences of Mothers of Pre-Term Infants* (London: National Childbirth Trust).

Thorpe, K., Golding, J., MacGillivray, I. and Greenwood R. (1991) 'Comparison of Prevalence of Depression in Mothers of Twins and Mothers of Singletons.' *British Medical Journal* **302**: 875–8.

Chapter 8

When a Baby Dies

Whilst it is customary to point out that all losses carry within them the potential for personal growth, the benefits of grief are not immediately apparent to people who have been bereaved. The circumstances surrounding the death of a baby would appear to indicate that parents will require a great deal of support if this potential is to be realized.

(Littlewood, 1996, p. 56)

This chapter is concerned with the range of experiences that mothers may undergo when a baby dies. Obviously, all of these experiences of loss are associated with intense maternal distress. The first part of the chapter commences with a discussion of the process of grief in general, and the second shows how the death of a baby is highly likely to be associated with complications arising during the process of grief. The third part of the chapter considers the impact that the death of a baby before birth may have upon his or her mother. Consequently, miscarriage and abortion will be discussed here. The fourth part of the chapter is concerned with expected and unexpected stillbirth and considers recent changes in policy and practice in this area. The fifth part of the chapter focuses upon deaths occurring on neonatal units, and the sixth part of the chapter briefly considers the special needs of mothers who have lost a twin and are left with a surviving infant. The final part of the chapter considers the impact of the death of a baby upon future childbearing.

The process of grief in contemporary Western society

The process of grieving amongst the general adult population has been relatively well documented by numerous researchers and it is possible, despite the wide variation in individual experiences, to identify a very general pattern associated with uncomplicated grief (Littlewood, 1992a). The initial response following the death of a loved person is usually one of shock and disbelief. However, despite an apparent inability to comprehend the loss, the person may suffer from outbursts of intense emotion, for example panic, sobbing or irrational anger.

The person goes on to experience an intense physical, emotional and cognitive reaction to the loss. The bereaved person longs for the return of the dead person and appears to be completely preoccupied by his or her image. Events immediately preceding the death are obsessively reviewed in an often abortive attempt to understand what has happened. Self-reproach for having caused, or failed to prevent, the death is often present, and anger, directed at self or others, is a frequently cited component of grief. Dreams and vivid hallucinations may occur, and a period of social withdrawal frequently accompanies this intense preoccupation with the dead person.

Following, or interspersed with, these experiences are feelings of apathy, fatigue and despair. Difficulty in concentration and disrupted sleeping patterns are commonly reported and thoughts of suicide are sometimes present. Eventually, episodes of relative normality occur for progressively longer periods of time, and episodes of grief decrease in frequency. The general consensus of researchers in the area would indicate that the whole process may take up to 2 years to progress to a point at which 'pangs' of grief are relatively self-contained and occur as occasional episodes. However, Raphael (1984) indicates that the deaths of children in general are often associated with what she calls 'shadow grief' in which the parents project the dead child's expected developmental path into the future and experience pangs of grief at, for example, the time when the dead child would have been expected to start school.

Descriptions of complicated grief are not uncommon, and these descriptions may be loosely gathered under three headings: delayed grief, chronic grief, and absent or distorted grief. Delayed grief occurs when the recognition of the loss is postponed. Typically, grief is experienced with particular severity at a later date. Chronic grief is associated with instances in which the expected range of reactions are present but the bereaved person does not recover from them. Raphael (1984) has suggested that in distorted reactions to bereavement, one aspect of grief is emphasised and others often suppressed. She further suggests that the two common patterns are extreme expressions of either anger or guilt. The apparent absence of grief has also been noted, and Bowlby (1969) has suggested that, whilst grief may be absent, other bereavement-related problems are usually present.

Whilst there have been many researchers who have documented complications that may arise during the process of grieving, Worden (1992) usefully groups the relevant risk factors under five headings: relational, historical, circumstantial, personality and social. Unfortunately, the death of a baby is associated with difficulties relevant to at least three of these headings: the relational, the circumstantial and the social.

In particular, narcissistic relationships in which the deceased represents an extension of the self have been found by Worden (1992) to be associated with complications arising during the grieving process. Furthermore, the likely circumstances surrounding the death of a baby, that is, the uncertainty (Lazare, 1979), the absence of a body (Simpson, 1979) and the unanticipated and untimely nature of the death (Parkes, 1972), have all been associated with complicated grief. Finally, losses that are socially unspeakable or socially negated (Lazare, 1979) and the absence of social support networks (Vachon *et al.*, 1982) have also been identified as contributing to complications arising during the process of grief. Unfortunately, to a greater or lesser extent, all of these problems are associated with the death of a baby.

Bereavement at the time of childbirth

The very nature of the relationship between parents and babies who die makes the nature of the loss more difficult to cope with. Raphael (1984) suggests that parents commit themselves to a baby in the hope that the baby will eventually gratify their own unfulfilled hopes and dreams. Thus, the baby may come to represent not only a physical, but also a psychological extension of the parents (Rando, 1986). These narcissistic expectations are obviously dashed if the baby should die and the mother may be left grieving not only for a baby but for a part of herself that may be seen to be indistinguishable from her child (Peretz, 1970).

Furthermore, Borg and Lasker (1982) suggest that the sheer intensity of the mother's feelings of grief may induce fear in the mother because the strength of her feelings does not match any tangible contact with the baby. Consequently, it is often difficult for the mother to understand exactly why she is so upset over a baby she barely knew. However, it is not the intensity of feelings of grief but the sheer complexity of them that may cause difficulties. Hutchins (1986) summarises these difficulties in terms of trying to say 'hello and goodbye' at the same time. This difficulty may account for some parental experiences of temporary 'euphoria' following seeing the body of their baby. For example, a father described ordering flowers for the funeral immediately after viewing his daughter's body in the following way:

> I don't know if what happened in the florists can be explained or not but it was very unusual. We walked in feeling on air... we were laughing and joking... and generally gave the impression that we were ordering flowers for a party rather than a funeral.
>
> *(Littlewood, 1992b, p. 4)*

As Nichols (1984) points out, the very intimacy of the parents' relationship with their baby makes the loss difficult to talk about – the hopes and dreams were essentially personal ones and may not be easy to either identify or share with other people.

Lewis and Bourne (1989) attribute maternal difficulty in accepting the loss of a baby to the uncertain and bewildering circumstances in which the death occurs; the mother may 'half know' of the death but can scarcely, owing to the unexpected nature of the event, bring herself to believe it. Lewis and Bourne liken the situation to that following 'missing, presumed dead' verdicts, situations in which complicated grief frequently occur (Lazare, 1979). For example:

> They'd told me he was dead but I just didn't believe it. The midwife said that I could have strong pain relief during labour because nothing I did would hurt the baby. I didn't have any pain relief, I wanted it to hurt because I thought that if it hurt he would be all right. When he was born, all I can remember thinking was please, please, don't let him be dead.
>
> *(Littlewood, 1992a, p. 123)*

The death of a baby is clearly both unexpected and untimely and both of these factors have been associated with complicated grief (Parkes, 1972). Kellner and Lake (1986) suggest that this exacerbates maternal feelings of confusion and loss of control. Mander (1994) indicates that 'survivor guilt' may be present, and feelings concerning 'it should have been me' further increase the woman's distress and confusion.

Lack of tangible memories may also leave her wondering why she is experiencing grief. Obviously, the adoption of the Stillbirth and Neonatal Death Society (SANDS) guidelines go some way to minimising these circumstantial factors, which are now well documented as being distressing and confusing. However, another circumstantial factor that affects the process of grief is age. A woman who bears children is usually young, and in contemporary society young people are rarely confronted by death or grief (Littlewood, 1992). Consequently, young people find these issues particularly difficult to cope with. Cooper (1980) points out that young parents tend to respond with anger and outrage over the death of a baby, and these responses are thought to bode ill in respect of the grieving process (Raphael, 1984).

Social support also proves difficult following the death of a baby. At one level, the meaning of the pregnancy is unique to the mother, and to a greater or lesser extent the father, but the meaning of such a loss is essentially hidden from others, and the mother may feel particularly isolated (Rando, 1986; Lewis and Bourne, 1989).

In terms of the wider society, the relatively infrequent deaths of babies are shrouded in secrecy (Borg and Lasker, 1982). Consequently, the mother may feel irrationally ashamed about her loss and be unwilling to speak about it. Furthermore, since the baby's death occurred in hospital, many people in the general community may treat the baby as a 'non-person' and trivialise the loss (Nichols, 1984). In an early piece of work, Bourne (1968) showed that GPs were extremely reluctant to even remember anything about a woman who had experienced a stillbirth; again, this type of avoidance has been shown further to complicate the process of grieving amongst the general population (Lazare, 1979).

Overall, the elements of lack of anticipation, difficulty in accepting the loss and lack of social support would all seem to combine to make the death of a baby uniquely difficult to cope with.

The death of a baby before birth

The contemporary debates surrounding the impact of miscarriage upon women are relatively recent. As Mander (1994) has suggested, miscarriage was traditionally disregarded in terms of it being a source of maternal distress. Mander suggests three main reasons for such disregard:

- The non-visibility and, therefore, non-recognition of the pregnancy and its loss;
- An assumption that 'quickening' was highly significant in terms of the development of the mother–baby relationship. Consequently, it was assumed that earlier losses were less meaningful;

- Limited knowledge concerning the emotional processes associated with early pregnancy. Consequently, it was assumed that the shorter the gestation period, the less emotional investment on behalf of the mother there was likely to be.

In terms of frequency, miscarriage is one of the most common losses associated with pregnancy. Clinically recognised miscarriages are estimated to occur in approximately one third of all pregnancies (Bansen and Stevens, 1992). However, as Oakley et al. (1990) have indicated, the loss of biological pregnancies may be much higher. The relative frequency of miscarriage has led some researchers (for example, Roberts 1989) to regard it as an unremarkable event. However, recent research has indicated that, at least for some women, miscarriage is a highly distressing event. In a relatively early piece of research, Peppers and Knapp (1980) found little difference, in terms of grief, between miscarriage, stillbirth and neonatal death. Furthermore, Friedman and Garth (1989), in a North American study utilising the Present State Examination, found that at 4 weeks after a miscarriage, 48 per cent of the women in their sample could be classified as psychiatric 'cases'. The distress that Friedman and Garth identified was largely of a depressive nature and was correlated with previous experience of miscarriage rather than childlessness. In a later study, Bansen and Stevens (1992) interviewed women who had miscarried a wanted first baby and found that, 2–5 months after the miscarriage, anger, guilt and fear about future childbearing were still present.

In these circumstances, well-meaning attempts at comfort involving miscarriage being portrayed as 'nature's way of preventing something worse' are likely to be ill-received (Iles, 1989). It seems reasonable to suggest that women's experience of miscarriage will vary due to a number of factors, for example:

- Whether the woman was aware that she was pregnant;
- Whether the woman wanted to be pregnant;
- Whether the woman wanted to be pregnant but had a history of previous miscarriages.

The above might all be expected to play a part in the woman's interpretation of her loss. Consequently, Worden (1992) advises caution over assumptions concerning the meaning of a pregnancy and its loss. Clearly, for some women, a miscarriage can be an absolute tragedy, but for others, the loss may be judged to be less severe. Certainly, Bourne and Lewis's (1991) observations regarding miscarriage being 'magnified into a catastrophe' may be premature, precisely because, for some women, miscarriage may already be a catastrophe.

The voluntary termination of pregnancy is also beset by debates concerning the impact that the experience will have upon the mother of the unborn child. Neustatter and Newson (1986) identify the range of women's experiences following voluntary termination of pregnancy. According to Neustatter and Newson, depending upon the woman's circumstances, these can range from relief to grief.

However, the issue of voluntary termination of pregnancy is a highly contentious one, and Marck (1994) has argued that the voices of pregnant women are silenced by the heat of this particular moral debate. She identifies the importance of seeking an understanding of the individual woman's appraisal of her own situation and points out that this appraisal may reflect many personal issues and life experiences that may not be directly connected to the pregnancy. However, Marck also suggests that reactions to women who wish to have their pregnancies terminated are at best often unhelpful, and at worst downright hostile. For example:

And she talked about physical pain – grabbing, pulling, taking her insides out. And she talked of humiliation and embarrassment, shame strong enough to keep the full nature of the pain from her consciousness until after she left the operating room, the room full of strangers looking at her with her legs up in the air, her most private body exposed. Katherine knew she could not undergo such an experience again. Many nurses and physicians have heard more than one colleague express the notion that being forced to undergo an abortion without adequate anaesthetic ensured that a woman would 'learn her lesson'. Katherine has experienced this belief that 'bad' women need to be 'taught a lesson' all of her life, starting with her own father.

(Marck, 1994, p. 129)

Blatantly vicious misogyny aside, the desire to 'teach lessons', benign or otherwise, is relatively well documented in instances of voluntary termination of pregnancy. For example:

People often ask why we don't counsel girls to have their babies and get them adopted, as a way of preventing them going through the trauma of abortion and also to help offset the shortage of babies for adoption. Well, very, very few girls feel they could go through with that. Certainly that is how 18 year old Cathy felt:

'I got a pregnancy test done and when I broke down at the positive result, the nurse suggested I should have it adopted. She said that it was the right thing to do, that I would feel better than if I got rid of it...'

(Neustatter and Newson, 1986, pp. 54–55)

151

However, as we have shown in Chapter 7, it is highly questionable whether relinquishment is less traumatic than voluntary termination of a pregnancy for the mother involved. Nevertheless, Marck's (1994) point concerning the voluntary termination of pregnancy being associated with advice concerned with 'doing' something about the pregnancy, rather than enquiries about how the woman 'feels' about her pregnancy, would appear to be confirmed by Cathy's experience.

Mander (1994) is relatively optimistic concerning grief associated with the voluntary termination of pregnancy. She estimates that only 5 per cent of women will go on to experience grief in these circumstances. However, the situation regarding the voluntary termination of a pregnancy for fetal abnormality probably has a different impact upon the woman involved when compared with other reasons for the voluntary termination of a pregnancy.

Iles (1989) has suggested six reasons why termination for fetal abnormality is associated with emotions other than relief:

- It is more likely that a wanted pregnancy is being terminated.
- A late termination is more likely to be known about by others and therefore more likely to provoke unsolicited advice from a larger group of people than would an early termination. Also, the labour associated with a late termination is longer and more distressing.
- Impairments that are not incompatible with life produce guilt in a mother who opts for termination.
- Fear of, or actual risk of, recurrence may threaten future childbearing.
- In older mothers, the chances of successfully completing a subsequent pregnancy may be diminishing.
- Perceptions of failure to achieve a 'normal' pregnancy and delivery may compound the guilt associated with opting for a termination of the pregnancy.

Lawrence (1989) found that 75 per cent of mothers who had undergone a termination of pregnancy for fetal abnormality experienced acute grief, and 21 per cent required psychiatric help following their termination. Iles (1989), utilising the Present State Examination, identified 39 per cent of the women in her sample as being psychiatric 'cases'. Iles also found that the mother's experience was more severe if the abnormality was non-life threatening and/or the termination occurred particularly late in the pregnancy. However,

Iles also found that reported distress fell to that of the general population at a 6-month follow-up interview after the loss.

Clearly, the experiences of women who have undergone miscarriage or voluntary abortion are variable. It is in these circumstances that both authors share the hope expressed by Marck:

> It is my hope that all caregivers regardless of personal values... will come to value the voices of women who seek their care.
>
> *(Marck, 1994, p. 136)*

Unfortunately, maternal experiences of the birth of a stillborn baby show considerably less variation, and the experience is frequently one of devastation.

Stillbirth: when a baby dies at or around the time of birth

Up until approximately 15 years ago, the death of a baby at or around the time of birth was subject to what has been termed 'rugby tackle management' (Mander, 1994). According to Mander, 'rugby tackle management' involved a combination of the following five courses of action:

- Remove the dead baby from the room as quickly as possible (hence the term 'rugby tackle management', to emphasise the speed and method by which this manoeuvre was achieved.)
- Discourage parents from seeing the baby.
- Discourage the parents from communicating about the baby.
- Encourage the parents to forget about the loss and to concentrate upon conceiving another baby.
- Institutional disposal of the baby's body, often in an unmarked grave.

The full impact of such well-meaning but misguided attempts at 'management' were often long term. For example:

> My mother took him and wrapped him in his shawl. She had him, she was the other side of the bedroom door with him and the doctor wouldn't let her in. He said it was better if I didn't see him. I'll regret that until the day I die. I couldn't have any more you see and I never even saw him. My mother said he was beautiful.
>
> *(Littlewood, 1992b, p. 4)*

This particular comment was made by a woman during an interview concerning her husband's death. She was 84 years old and her baby had died 60 years prior to her comments.

In one of the relatively early arguments for changing professional practice, Lewis summarised the impact of such practice in the following way:

> This avoidance by the helping professionals extends into the neglect of the study of the effect of stillbirth on the mother and the family. There is a conspiracy of silence. We seem unwilling to come to terms with the fact that it is a tragedy which can seriously affect the mental health of the bereaved mother and her family. After the failure to mourn, mothers can have psychotic breakdowns or there can be severe mental difficulties. Children born before or after a stillbirth where there has been a failure to mourn a stillbirth can have severe emotional difficulties.
>
> *(Lewis, 1979, p. 303)*

However, Morris (1988) showed how, in less than a decade, practice had radically changed in some areas:

> The routine photography of all stillborn and now even miscarriages, and practices such as giving parents the baby's name tag, lock of hair or other memento shows how much progress has been made.
>
> *(Morris, 1988, p. 871)*

Changes in professional practice were supported by self-help initiatives developed by parents. In 1992 the SANDS guidelines were given official endorsement in England and Wales by a central government committee:

> We recommend that the guidelines drawn up for SANDS should form the basis for training of all professionals and managers involved in maternity care for dealing with bereavement. All units should ensure that such training is given to staff in a properly designed way.
>
> *(Winterton Report, 1992, p. 120)*

The committee's overall conclusions are also of interest:

> We conclude that the evidence highlighted the over-arching need for professionals to take account of best practice in this area and to formulate coherent and sensitive policies to address the needs of parents and families who experience miscarriage, stillbirth and neonatal death.
>
> *(Winterton Report, 1992, p. 120)*

Essentially this adoption of the SANDS guidelines represented a reversal of the previous mode of 'management.' Far from being encouraged to forget, parents are now encouraged to remember their baby. Mementoes are made available and parents are encouraged to talk openly about their loss. Furthermore, parents frequently view the body of their baby and dispose of the body with ritual. However, the death of a child around the time of birth remains a profoundly painful experience, and best practice may not always be taken into account. For example:

> I was left holding Hesther while people, as it seemed to me, backed off into the corners of the room. I spoke to her and cried with her... I held out my hand towards the retreating figures and asked for help. They retreated further and further away.
>
> *(Fairbairn, 1992, p. 290)*

Whilst the avoidance of both people who are dying and their relatives is an extremely common experience reported by people who have been bereaved (Littlewood, 1992a), this particular example of it had unfortunate consequences for the father in question because eventually, in a state of confusion and considerable emotional distress, he left his baby to be with his wife and retrospectively:

> wondered what possessed me to let my baby die in a room full of strangers while I ran off and hid from her.
>
> *(Fairbairn, 1992, p. 291)*

Stillbirth is, mercifully, a rare occurrence. However, when it does occur, what is expected to be a joyful event turns into a tragedy that is typically unexpected by the mother and those in attendance. Kirkley-Best and Kellner (1982), in their review of the area, indicate that the most common circumstances surrounding stillbirth are those in which the baby is viable until labour. Even in cases where there is forewarning of the death, these authors suggest that this may be met with a lack of comprehension on the part of the parents. Consequently, parental reaction to the occurrence of a stillbirth may be similar in both instances.

Whilst in general circumstances, a period of time in which to anticipate that a death will occur has been argued to be beneficial to those about to be bereaved, Jolly (1987) suggests that the mother carrying a dead baby may feel like a 'living coffin'. Alternatively, Hutchins (1986) argues that the mother may beneficially begin anticipatory grief in the antenatal period, but, as Grubb (1976) and Kish (1978) point out, the situation is complicated because profound disturbances of body image featuring uncleanliness and horror may be present.

For various reasons, some medical and some psychological, the induction of labour is usually recommended in these cases, and Dyer

(1992) suggests that waiting for a day or two may better enable the mother to orientated herself to the loss. However, whilst more research clearly needs to be conducted in this area, the overall evidence would indicate that the woman may persist in 'hoping for the best'. Furthermore, Mander (1994) indicates that the mother may not be alone with her hopes:

> There is a moment at the birth when everyone who is present, the parents and the staff, see that the baby has been born and hope against hope that the baby is going to cry. I know that it's quite illogical, but you still hope. And it is not until that moment when we all realise that the baby really is dead, that we all finally realise it is so.
>
> *(Mander, 1994, p. 39)*

In cases of unexpected stillbirth, shock remains the primary feature (Hutchins, 1986), and initial reactions appear to be minimal (Bourne, 1978). However, Wolff *et al.* (1970) noted a tendency towards anger for up to 3 years after the event. These researchers also noted a tendency for parents to either seek solace in another child or to develop a fear of pregnancy and childbirth. Culberg (1971) conducted a similar study and found that approximately one third of mothers were experiencing symptoms that were severe enough to warrant the diagnosis of a psychiatric illness.

Alternatively, Cooper (1980) indicated that the couples in her study perceived the stillbirth as a threat to their integrity or a medical accident to be exposed, rather than as a loss to be mourned. In this sense, the reactions would appear to be similar to the reactions of parents who have lost children in disasters. As Hodgkinson has indicated:

> Following the Zeebrugge disaster, parents who had lost adult children, for whom no compensation was indicated in British law, banded together to form the Herald Families Association. They were enraged that they were symbolically denied recognition that they had been bereaved. Their avowed aim was to see the prosecution of the ferry operator for negligence and the institution of safer ferry standards. It remains to be seen whether this channelling of anger will prove an aid or block to resolution.
>
> *(Hodgkinson, 1989, pp. 353–354)*

Whilst there is an urgent need for more research in the area of long-term adjustment to stillbirth, it seems reasonable to suggest that the factors surrounding stillbirth may make the process of grief painfully difficult and complicated.

Neonatal death

Babies are admitted to NNUs when a health problem has either been recognised or is likely to arise. Loss is a predominant theme amongst the parents of such babies, irrespective of whether or not their baby dies. Whilst the losses associated with admission to an NNU have been addressed in Chapter 7, Benfield *et al.* (1978) have argued that grieving a baby who has died on a NNU is a highly individual experience but that parental concerns include anger, guilt, disbelief and a sense of unreality. Whilst grief is never easy, Lewis and Bourne (1989) have suggested that neonatal death is not so shocking as stillbirth because the parents have had time to be with their baby and therefore find it easier to attribute personhood to him or her. Furthermore, the presence of the staff on the NNU who have all been committed to the care of the baby may, to a certain extent, help the parents to validate the baby's social existence (Littlewood, 1992b).

Alternatively, helplessly watching a futile struggle for survival may serve to sharpen an already deeply felt distress. For example:

At the birth of her child Ms W felt that if he was going to have to be kept alive artificially, then it was better that he should die. However, when she saw her son he looked better than she expected and efforts were made. By the third day of his life Ms W felt differently and desperately hoped that her son would survive. However, she was told that there was no hope of his recovery and that the machines were to be switched off. Ms W felt that the fact that her son had struggled to survive made his personality seem that much stronger, so the decision to let him die was much harder to take... Ms W remembered feeling shattered when the death finally occurred.

(Littlewood, 1992b, pp. 127–128)

Also, anticipatory loss may lead parents to feel uncertain about forming a relationship with an ill baby (Kennell and Klaus, 1982). This may, paradoxically, result in guilt if the baby subsequently dies.

Furthermore, the tendency for the broader community to avoid or minimise the extent of a loss when a baby dies on an NNU would appear to be comparable to communal reactions, or rather more accurately the lack of them, to a stillbirth (Helmrath and Steinitz, 1978). Nichols (1984) attributes most of the problems encountered by the parents of dying newborns to discounted grief and negated death. Again, more research is required in order to clarify these issues.

The death of a twin

As Thorpe *et al.* (1991) have indicated, the death of an infant and the bereavement that follows may be unique in the case of twins. Where there is a surviving twin, the distressed mother has the demands of a new baby, a baby that may remind her of the baby she has lost, to cope with during her bereavement (Lewis and Bryan, 1988).

In addition, the mother may be perceived as 'still having a baby', and her need for sympathy and support over her loss may go unnoticed (Green, 1990). In Thorpe *et al.*'s (1991) study, the mothers who had lost one twin had the highest malaise scores 1 year after the birth compared with mothers of surviving twins and single babies. However, it must be said that mothers who had lost both twins or a single baby were not followed up, so no comparative data of this nature were available. Nevertheless, it seems reasonable to suggest that bereavement coupled with the demands of a new baby might make the death of one twin a particularly difficult loss to cope with.

Future childbearing

Whilst the decision to embark upon another pregnancy following a stillbirth or neonatal death is highly individual (Wolff *et al.*, 1970), an urgent desire for another pregnancy at a relatively early stage of grieving is, in itself, believed further to complicate the process of grief. Leon (1990) interprets the prevalence and urgency of such desires in terms of the mother's damaged self-esteem and argues that a subsequent successful pregnancy becomes the only route by which the woman believes she will regain her equilibrium.

However, whilst Lewis and Bourne (1989) agree that a subsequent pregnancy may shorten grief, they indicate that the effect is temporary and argue that grief may re-emerge either at the time of the subsequent birth or at some unforeseeable time in the future. Whilst the longer-term implications are difficult to foresee and research, Mander feels confident enough to assert that, at least in the short term:

> we may be certain that a mother who hurries or is hurried into another pregnancy is likely to find the experience unpleasant or even traumatic.
>
> *(Mander, 1994, p. 185)*

However, the desire to have a child may be particularly strong, and whilst a subsequent pregnancy may well be indicative of problems associated with grief, this may not always be the case. Nevertheless, health-care professionals need to be aware of the special needs that a woman who has lost a child and is embarking upon a subsequent pregnancy may have.

Conclusion

This chapter has been concerned with the nature of the grieving process following the death of a baby. It has been suggested that recent changes in practice may, given the generic knowledge concerning the process of grief, go some way to ameliorating maternal distress. Contemporary practice should mitigate the confusion and sense of unreality that are inevitably present following the death of a baby. In short, the available evidence would suggest that we now have enough knowledge to avoid, unwittingly or otherwise, making things worse. However, actual research concerning the impact of the introduction of, for example, the SANDS guidelines is long overdue.

The death of a baby is often a tragedy for the mother and the evidence would indicate that the lack of availability of support in the community should give cause for concern since the factors surrounding the death of a child at, or around the time of, birth are frequently those which are known to complicate the process of grief amongst the adult population in general. Voluntary termination for fetal abnormality would appear to be particularly distressing, and although the impact of the experience of miscarriage may be variable, it is clear that miscarriage may be an extremely traumatic and distressing experience for some women. Stillbirth would appear to be associated with anger and outrage to a greater extent than other deaths. However, this is another area that would benefit from future research.

Alternatively, deaths that occur on neonatal units may be associated with ambivalence and guilt that may cause mothers additional distress. Further investigation is needed to clarify these issues.

Despite the fact, outside miscarriage, of the rarity of the loss of a baby, such a loss may represent a potential disaster for the mother. Consequently, we urgently need to further our understanding of the aftermath, in both the short and the long term, of such a loss. Many, if not most, women whose baby dies go on to have other children, and the evidence would suggest that they may need a great deal of care, understanding and support.

Whilst it is customary to point out that all losses carry within them the potential for personal growth, the benefits of grief are by no means immediately apparent to mothers who have been bereaved. The very circumstances surrounding the death of a baby would appear to indicate that mothers will require a great deal of support if this potential is to be realised.

Unfortunately, bereavement is one of many losses associated with maternal distress. The help available for other, less catastrophic but nevertheless distressing, forms of maternal distress and depression is the subject of the final chapter.

References

Bansen, S. S. and Stevens, M. A. (1992) 'Women's Experience of Miscarriage in Early Pregnancy.' *Journal of Nurse Midwifery* **37**(2): 84–90.

Benfield, G., Lieb, S. and Volman, J. (1978) 'Grief Response of Parents to Neonatal Death and Parent Participation in Deciding Care.' *Paediatrics* **62**:171–7.

Borg, A. and Lasker, J. (1982) *When Pregnancy Fails* (London: Routledge).

Bourne, S. (1968) 'The Psychological Effects of Stillbirth on Women and their Doctors.' *Journal of the Royal College of General Practitioners* **16**:103–12.

Bourne, S. (1978) 'Coping with Perinatal Death.' *Midwife, Health Visitor and Community Nurse* February: 59–62.

Bourne, S. and Lewis, E. (1991) 'Perinatal Bereavement: A Milestone and Some New Dangers.' *British Medical Journal* **302**: 1167–8.

Bowlby, J. (1969) *Attachment and Loss*, vol. 1 (London: Hogarth Press).

Cooper, J. D. (1980) 'Parental Reactions to Stillbirth.' *British Journal of Social Work* **10**: 55–69.

Culberg, J. (1971) 'Mental Reactions of Women to Perinatal Death.' *Proceedings of the Third Congress of Psychosomatic Medicine, Obstetrics and Gynaecology* (Basel: Karger).

Dyer, M. (1992) 'Stillborn – Still Precious.' *MIDIRS Digest* **2**(2): 341–4.

Fairbairn, G. (1992) 'When a Baby Dies – A Father's View.' In Dickenson, D. and Johnson, M. (eds) *Death, Dying and Bereavement* (London: Sage).

Friedman, T. and Garth, D. (1989) 'The Psychiatric Consequences of Spontaneous Abortion.' *British Journal of Psychiatry* **155**: 810–3.

Green, J. (1990) 'Calming or Harming? A Clinical Review of Psychological Effects of Fetal Diagnosis of Pregnant Women.' Occasional Papers, second series no. 2 (London: Galton Institute).

Grubb, C. A. (1976) 'Body Image Concerns of a Multipara in the Situation of Intrauterine Fetal Death.' *Maternal Child Nursing* **5**: 93.

Helmrath, T. A. and Steinitz, E. M. (1978) 'Death of an Infant: Parent Grieving and the Failure of Social Support.' In Rando, T. A. (ed.) *Parental Loss of a Child* (Champaign, IL: Research Press).

Hodgkinson, P. E. (1989) 'Technological Disaster – Survival and Bereavement.' *Social Sciences and Medicine* **55**: 29–34.

Hutchins, S. H. (1986) 'Stillbirth.' In Rando, T. A. (ed.) *Parental Loss of a Child* (Champaign, IL: Research Press).

Iles, S. (1989) 'The Loss of Early Pregnancy.' In Oates, M. R. (ed.) *Psychological Aspects of Obstetrics and Gynaecology* (London: Baillière Tindall).

Jolly, J. (1987) *Missed Beginning* (London: Austen Cornish).

Kellner, K. R. and Lake, M. (1989) 'Grief Counselling.' In Knuppel, R. A. and Drukker, J. E. (eds) *High Risk Pregnancy* (Philadelphia: W. B. Saunders).

Kennell, J. H. and Klaus, M. H. (1982) 'Caring for the Parents of Premature Sick Infants.' In Klaus, M. H. and Kennell, J. H. (eds) *Parent Infant Bonding*, 2nd edn (St Louis: C. V. Mosby).

Kirkley-Best, E. and Kellner, K. (1982) 'The Forgotten Grief: A Review of the Psychology of Stillbirth.' *American Journal of Orthopsychiatry* 52: 20–9.

Kish, G. (1978) 'Notes on C. Grubb's Body Image Concerns of a Multipara in the Situation of Intrauterine Fetal Death.' *Maternal Child Nursing* 7: 11.

Lawrence, K. M. (1989) 'Sequelae and Support for Termination carried out for Fetal Malformation.' In van Hall, E. V. and Everaerd, W. (eds) *The Freeman: Women's Health in the 1990s* (Carnforth: Parthenon).

Lazare, A. (1979) 'Unresolved Grief.' In Lazare, A. (ed.) *Outpatient Psychiatry: Diagnosis and Treatment* (Baltimore: Williams and Wilkins).

Leon, I. G. (1990) *When a Baby Dies: Psychotherapy for Pregnancy and Newborn Loss* (London: Yale University Press).

Lewis, E. (1979) 'Mourning by the Family after a Stillbirth or Neonatal Death.' *Archives of Disease in Childhood* 55: 303–6.

Lewis, E. and Bourne, S. (1989) 'Perinatal Death.' In Oates, M. (ed.), *Psychological Aspects of Obstetrics and Gynaecology* (London: Baillière Tindall).

Lewis, E. and Bryan E. M. (1988) 'Management of Perinatal Loss of a Twin.' *British Medical Journal* 297: 1321–2.

Littlewood, J. (1992a) *Aspects of Grief: Bereavement in Adult Life* (London: Routledge).

Littlewood, J. (1992b) A Comparison of Maternal Experiences of Stillbirth and Neonatal Death.' Unpublished paper presented to the Annual Conference of the Society for Reproductive and Infant Psychology, Glasgow, September.

Littlewood, J. (1996) 'Stillbirth and Neonatal Death'. In Niven, C. A. and Walker, A. (eds) *Conception, Pregnancy and Birth*, vol. 2 of *The Psychology of Reproduction* (Oxford: Butterworth-Heinemann).

Mander, R. (1994) *Loss and Bereavement in Childbearing* (London: Blackwell Scientific).

Marck, P. B. (1994) 'Unexpected Pregnancy: The Unchartered Land of Women's Experience.' In Field, P. A. and Marck, P. B. (eds) *Uncertain Motherhood: Negotiating the Risks of the Childbearing Years* (London: Sage Publications).

Morris, D. (1988) 'Management of Perinatal Bereavement.' *Archives of Disease in Childhood* 63: 870–2.

Neustatter, A. and Newson, G. (1986) *Mixed Feelings: The Experience of Abortion* (London: Pluto Press).

Nichols, J. A. (1984) 'Illegitimate Mourners.' In Symposium on Children and Death Perspectives and Challenges, Akron, OH, September.

Oakley, A., McPherson, A. and Roberts, H. (1990) *Miscarriage* (London: Penguin Books).

Parkes, C. M. (1972) *Bereavement* (New York: International Universal Press).

Peppers, L. G. and Knapp, R. J. (1980) 'Maternal Reactions to Involuntary Fetal/Infant Death.' *Psychiatry* **43**: 155–9.

Peretz, D. (1970) 'Reactions to Loss.' In Schoenberg, B., Karr, D., Peretz, D. and Kutsher, A. H. (eds) *Loss and Grief: Psychological Management in Medical Practice* (Columbia: Columbia University Press).

Rando, T. A. (ed.) (1986) *Parental Loss of a Child* (Champaign, IL: Research Press).

Raphael, B. (1994) *The Anatomy of Bereavement: A Handbook for the Caring Professions* (London: Unwin Hyman).

Roberts, H. (1989) 'A Baby or the Products of Conception: Lay and Professional Perspectives on Miscarriage.' In van Hall, E. V. and Everaerd, W. (eds) *The Freeman: Women's Health in the 1990s* (Carnforth: Parthenon).

Simpson, M. A. (1979) *The Facts of Death* (Englewood Cliffs, NJ: Prentice-Hall).

Thorpe, K., Golding, G., MacGillivray, I. and Greenwood. R. (1991) 'Comparison of Prevalence of Depression in Mothers of Twins and Mothers of Singletons.' *British Medical Journal* **302**: 875–8.

Vachon, M. L. S., Sheldon, A. R., Lancee, S. L. *et al.* (1982) 'Correlates of Enduring Distress Patterns Following Bereavement: Social Network Life Situation and Personality.' *Psychological Medicine* **12**: 783–8.

Winterton Report (1992) *Health Committee Second Report on the Maternity Services*, vol. 1 (London: HMSO).

Wolff, J. R., Nielson, P. E. and Schiller, P. (1970) 'The Emotional Reaction to a Stillbirth.' *American Journal of Obstetrics and Gynecology* **108**: 73–7.

Worden, J. W. (1992) *Grief Counselling and Grief Therapy: A Handbook for the Mental Health Practitioner*, 2nd edn (London: Routledge).

Chapter 9

Helping Women Who Become Distressed and/or Depressed Following Childbirth

Only relatively recently has motherhood become a lonely condition, when responsibility for the sole care of another human being, the baby, may be experienced as overwhelming and burdensome in its isolation.

(Ashurst and Hall, 1989, p. 155)

So far, we have concentrated on looking at different theories of post-natal depression and what might constitute potential causes of maternal distress. This has entailed looking at cultural and social attitudes to motherhood and medical and social attitudes towards mental illness in women. Crucial to this area is the provision of maternity services and the underlying philosophy behind maternity care. The final chapters have looked at women's own experiences and the differing circumstances of these experiences.

But what support is available for women once distress or depression is established? As we have already argued, the different approaches and theoretical arguments in this area are of little consequence to women undergoing distressing experiences post-childbirth if there is no support or help available. Access to support and help vary as much as the theories behind the causes of depression and distress. As the causes of each woman's depression or distress are likely to be different, it would make sense that the provision of support and treatment should also be individualised to a woman's specific needs. However, as we have previously indicated, detection rates do not actually reflect rates of depression/distress. Taylor *et al.* (1994) found in a study looking at the risk factors, identification and effects of postnatal depression that 80 per cent of women had neither sought nor received medical help. Taylor *et al.* suggest that women do not come forward because they do not realise that medical help is available. Only 20 per cent of the women in this small study had sought medical aid, and only 18 per cent had spoken to their health visitor.

It is possible that women would not wish to be identified as not coping with motherhood, as being perceived as inadequate. Holden's (1994) study of health visitor's use of the EPDS indicated that up to 60 per cent of health visitors not using the Scale were unaware that the women in their care were depressed. Clements (1995) attributes this to the possibility that women find it hard to tell health professionals that they are depressed. Cox (1986) found it ironic that, although women had regular contact with health professionals in the early puerperium, postnatal depression was rarely detected. Cox postulated that it is possible that some primary health-care workers, such as health visitors or midwives, may feel out of their depth with a perceived psychiatric disorder even if it was initially detected.

McIntosh (1993) examined women's help-seeking behaviours and their own perceptions of the cause of their depression. McIntosh looked at the experiences of 60 primiparous women and found that the majority of depressed women did not seek help from any sources and that, of the women studied, only 25 per cent consulted a health professional. The low levels of help-seeking behaviour were explained in terms of women's understanding of the causes of their depression, their difficulty in admitting that they were experiencing emotional difficulties and their perceptions of how appropriate available help was to their particular situation. McIntosh observed that women identified that they were too ashamed to seek help from close family and friends as they saw their emotional problems as signs of personal inadequacy and an admission of failure on their behalf. Again, in McIntosh's study, only 26 per cent of the women went to health professionals for help. The two main reasons for this were identified as follows. Firstly, professional help was not perceived as relevant to the women's understanding of their problems, and, secondly, there was a worry that admitting to emotional difficulties would result in them being labelled as mentally ill and therefore unfit mothers. Frequently, when professional help was sought, it was only as a last resort when the women were having difficulties with everyday functioning.

As already stated, facilities and access to support varies considerably across the country. Prettyman and Friedman (1991) compiled a survey of the then current provisions for inpatient care for mothers and their babies across England and Wales. With a response rate of

97 per cent of health authorities, Prettyman and Friedman established that only 19 per cent had facilities specifically for mothers and
babies, and in 21 districts (10 per cent of those who replied) there
was no provision at all for any degree of joint admission. When
considering the strength of the medical model of care in this area, the
provision of support and help would appear to be weak. In the 19 per
cent of districts that reported mother and baby facilities, just under
half the women were admitted under the care of a consultant with
no specified special interest in puerperal psychiatry. Prettyman and
Friedman did establish that the provision of such services was
deemed important, and 93 health authorities said that there were
plans either to review services or to establish mother and baby inpatient facilities. In some areas, the provision of such facilities would
appear to prove uneconomical in relation to the birth rate for that
area. Although the 'Health of the Nation' report (Department of
Health, 1993) has put mental health as high on its agenda, it would
be interesting to see how the plans reported to Prettyman and
Friedman (1991) have been effected by the economic climate of
hospital trust status to many psychiatric units across the country.

Access to voluntary organisations also varies across the
country, and women's ability to access these organisations and
groups may depend upon a number of factors such as publicity of
what is available, childcare facilities, distance to travel and availability of transport.

In the following section the types of professional help available will
be examined. This will include the professionals available, screening
tools, styles of treatment and types of facilities.

Professional input

Pregnancy and the early postnatal period are a time when most
women have heavy contact with health-care professionals, possibly
more so than at any other point in their lives.

Antenatally, the main contact will be with the midwife, GP and
obstetrician. Postnatally, contact will also include the health visitor,
whose role becomes more prominent, and the midwife who works
with women up to 28 days postnatally. Should emotional problems be
detected, other professionals available will include the psychiatrist,
psychiatric and community psychiatric nurses, social workers and
clinical psychologists.

Table 9.1 Ante- and postnatal contact with health professionals

Health professional	Type of contact
GP	Family care. Should know woman, potentially over a long period of time. May not have had much contact
Midwife/midwives	Main contact throughout pregnancy, labour and postnatal period. Ideally placed to build up good relationship, but the woman may meet many midwives and not get the chance to develop a relationship with any of them
Obstetrician	Most women book for care with a specific consultant but, unless there are difficulties with the pregnancy, will probably have very little contact. May have limited contact with junior doctors in hospital
Health visitor	Many women may meet their health visitor antenatally or already have had contact through previous children. The health visitor is often perceived as only being concerned with child development, but will get to know woman over a longer period of time and has a valuable role to play in support and detection
Psychiatrist	Women only referred to if there is a problem established. May or may not have a special interest in postpartum disorders. Facilities available will depend on area
Psychiatric nurse	Will be met when problem is established. Will be seen by women on an in or outpatient basis. Contact will depend on type of unit, methods of staffing units and specialty of staff
Community psychiatric nurse	Met in community setting. Visits to woman in own environment when problem established. Will provide counselling, support and assessment of medication. Again provision of care will depend upon local facilities and polices of care plus availability of community psychiatric nurse
Social workers	May meet antenatally, usually when a need is established. Can offer ongoing support, counselling and advice about benefits and housing issues. Availability depends on local facilities
Clinical psychologist	Will be met when need is established. May be hospital or community based, will provide counselling and support dependent on availability. Support can include, for example, family therapy and cognitive behavioural therapy. Can offer support to other professionals in establishing and monitoring services
Occupational therapist	Will be met as part of multidisciplinary psychiatric team. Organises group therapy, counselling and support plus stress management programmes

We have already seen that detection rates do not reflect the incidence of postnatal depression and distress, either through the inability of professionals to detect problems or because women are reluctant to seek help and face the possibility of being labelled as inadequate mothers. For those women who do come forward, what can the medical profession offer in terms of treatment and facilities?

The first admission of mother and babies to psychiatric units occurred in the early 1950s (Oates, 1988). The development of units was through the establishment either of special mother and baby units, or special facilities on general psychiatric wards. Lindsay and Pollard (1978) found that where joint admission of the mother and baby was possible, the recovery rate of the mother was more rapid and the rate of relapse reduced.

Riley (1995) has identified a number of problems with inpatient psychiatric facilities. The service can be quite expensive to staff, and, on an economic basis, can be argued not to represent the most efficient use of resources, many of the units having a low bed occupancy with intermittent demand. Inpatient care, even if it does include mother and baby facilities, can present certain difficulties for some women. Most health professionals would agree that women who present with serious mental health problems that could present a problem to themselves or their baby need inpatient care and support:

> No member of the multi-disciplinary team would suggest the management of the patient at home if the baby was involved in the psychotic process or if the mother was engaged in potentially hazardous behaviour towards the baby.
>
> *(Oates, 1988, p. 157)*

However, for other women, the admission as an inpatient presents certain problems. For multigravid women who are single parents or who are in a relationship and have older children, the disruption to the family may prove too much and they may resist admission to hospital. Inpatient admission may impose further disruption to a family that is already struggling to cope. The unit itself may not be situated locally as some women are admitted to regional units, and this may cause further stresses through travelling or isolation for the woman from her friends and relatives. Additionally, women who are already emotionally vulnerable may be further traumatised by an admission into a psychiatric unit that may also have other acutely disturbed clients, as the following quote from a 29-year-old woman, describing her resistance to being admitted to the local psychiatric unit, shows:

I could not bear the thought of being admitted to [named unit], it would have pushed me further over the edge. That would have represented the final straw, the confirmation that I was going totally mad. If I managed to stay out, then I had something to cling onto. But if I ended up in there then I felt I would just disintegrate.

Riley (1995) states that the ideal unit would be locally placed, although for areas of dispersed population this would prove difficult. The unit would have the facilities of a day hospital and day nursery. There should ideally be provision for inpatient care facilities for moderately disturbed women not requiring admission, which should include care for older children and babies, with appropriately trained staff. Facilities would be available to provide overnight stays for partners. Finally, Riley states that the ideal unit would also act as a resource centre and training unit.

Oates (1988) in Nottingham provides an example of a good alternative to hospital inpatient care. The Nottingham scheme evolved as an integrated community-orientated service for women with severe postnatal depression:

The philosophy of care is to achieve the bespoke management of an individual patient deploying the resources of the community, the family and the psychiatric team flexibly in order to preserve continuity of mother/infant relationship and to minimize the effects of maternal illness on other members of the family.

(Oates, 1988, p. 155)

Oates states that the aim of the integrated community service is to provide for the individual needs of each woman and her family. The role of the community psychiatric nurses would be to act as key workers in a multidisciplinary team. The philosophy of care incorporates seven basic principles: assessment, relief of symptoms, maternal autonomy and self-esteem, individuality, universality, realism and, finally, socialisation and group identity.

The initial principle of assessment entails a community psychiatric nurse assessing a potential client's home and social circumstances, what support is already available and what else would be needed to care for the woman in her own environment. The community psychiatric nurse, following assessment, would then be able to compile a management of care plan.

For a woman experiencing the distressing symptoms of depression, a priority of care would be the relief of symptoms. Relief would be obtained through the monitoring of medication and continuous assessment of the women's mental state. Home-based care can also be appropriate for women receiving ECT. The presence of the community psychiatric nurse would also allow space for one-to-one counselling and support.

In helping to develop maternal autonomy and self-esteem, the aim is also to facilitate a positive relationship between the mother and her baby. Any nursing care of the baby is preferably carried out in front of the mother so as not to undermine the woman's confidence in her childcare skills. Ideally, the role of the community psychiatric nurse is to support the women's partner and key relatives in aiding recovery of the woman's confidence levels.

In terms of individuality, the role of the key worker is to aid the woman in creating her own individual style of mothering. This creation of an individual mothering style may turn out to have very little similarity to the woman's own experience of mothering or her preconceived expectations and images.

Tying in with individuality and ideas of mothering are women's feelings of guilt at experiencing negative emotions towards their role as mother or towards the baby. It is common for women to feel guilty or abnormal for experiencing emotions such as anger, irritation or dislike. The hardest thing about these emotions is that they are largely unacknowledged and therefore individual women may not realise how common they actually are. The community psychiatric nurse is in an ideal position in Oates' scheme to reduce feelings of alienation by acknowledging the reality of these emotions and also how common they are.

This leads on to the principle of realism when a woman has unrealistic expectations of herself as a mother and often of what is normal infant behaviour. The established relationship of the nurse and the woman can open up issues in this area that can hopefully be backed up by the input of primary health-care workers such as the health visitor:

> Many of these mothers have idealized and unrealistic expectations of themselves and motherhood. The failure of both mother and baby to achieve these ideals leads to a feeling that the mother is inadequate and that the baby's essentially normal behaviour is a manifestation of her inadequacy.
>
> *(Oates, 1988, p. 156)*

The final stage in the principles of care process is the concept of socialisation and group identity. At this stage, when the key worker and woman feel it is appropriate, the woman is encouraged to obtain contact with local mother and toddler groups and, where available, professionally run support groups for women recovering from postnatal depression.

Oates feels that an integrated community service is a positive step in the care of women with postnatal depression, be it moderate or severe. However, this system of care is only appropriate when the woman has close relatives to offer support in the absence of the key worker. It also requires the back-up and resources of a specialist multidisciplinary team with access to a mother and baby unit. It is most appropriate where the potential client is within easy reach of these facilities, that is, is in an urban situation rather than a rural one.

Women themselves who were involved with the Nottingham scheme gave positive evaluations of its outcomes and perceived their recovery time as being quicker compared with any previous occasions of postnatal depression:

> The clinical recovery of those seventeen patients in the study who had been admitted for a previous episode of puerperal psychosis was the same with intensive home nursing. Interestingly most of these patients thought that they had recovered more quickly when they were managed at home with their second episode.
>
> *(Oates, 1988, p. 158)*

The Nottingham scheme has many positive outcomes, and the maintenance of the family unit within a community setting is a strong bonus. The role of the key worker is crucial in this. Oates states that the key worker input varied from 8 hours continuous daily nursing to care on alternate days. In the present economic climate, it is easy to wonder how such a labour-intensive scheme will fare and whether demand will outstrip supply.

The alternative to a community care service would be the provision of a day hospital facility. The provision of day care is seen as appropriate for women with moderately severe emotional problems. Again, Riley (1995) argues that this type of service might only be appropriate in an urban setting with a high population density. Perhaps the best known of the day hospital schemes is that currently operating in Stoke-on-Trent. The Charles Street Parent and Baby Day Unit in Stoke-on-Trent was fully established in 1988 after a specialised service was offered within a generic psychiatric hospital. Charles Street is more centrally placed and could offer nursery facilities. Staffing is again centered around a multidisciplinary team comprising consultant psychiatrist, unit manager, psychiatric nurses, occupational therapists, clinical assistants, nursery nurses, a clinical psychologist and administrative staff.

Each woman who was referred received an assessment interview and, in appropriate cases, an assessment with a psychiatrist. Ideally, women were asked to attend with their partner, if they had one. Women are allocated a key worker to coordinate a programme of care:

The key worker co-ordinates the care programme which is individually tailored and may include counselling as well as group activities.

(Cox, 1993, p. 711)

The women are encouraged to attend open groups, where experiences and feelings are expressed and the group members receive support from each other. Women at Charles Street also receive information about the symptomatology of postnatal depression, the range of treatments available and types of prevention, and sessions on stress management.

Assessment questionnaires by clients 1 year after Charles Street opened showed that women wanted their partners involved more, for them to attend a father's group and to have more involvement in therapy sessions. Women valued the deployment of key workers and use of home visits. Women also expressed the desire for increased information on childcare, diet, family management and health issues. Following the results of this evaluation, social activities were changed to make it easier for partners, and a group for women with older children was initiated.

Our experiences would suggest, however, that a day hospital with close links to a mother and baby unit, as well as a community specialist team is likely to provide an optimum service – as well as being a centre for education, research and development.

(Cox, 1993, p. 713)

Cox has also been heavily involved in the development of a screening test that would be readily acceptable to women, accessible to other health professionals and quick to administer. The EPDS has become the most widely used screening tool with postnatal depression and was validated in 1987 (Cox, 1987). The prevailing screening scales were considered to be inappropriate for use with postpartum women. Examples of depression screening scales include the Beck Depression Inventory (Beck *et al.*, 1961), Anxiety and Depression Self-report Scale (Bedford and Foulds, 1978) and the General Health

Questionnaire (Goldberg, 1972). Items that would increase the score on these questionnaires are commonplace for many women, both antenatally and postnatally. Problems can be specifically identified with items relating to change in sleeping patterns, tiredness, feeling off colour, and so on, all of which can be common in early pregnancy and the early postpartum period.

Holden (1994) states that research evidence would indicate that the EPDS is a reliable reflection of women's moods at the time of completion and an indicator of signs of depression in women. A specific advantage of this scale (see Appendix II) for postnatal depression is that it is a short ten-item questionnaire, making it easy to complete. Additionally, the EPDS does not require specialist knowledge to rate, so it can be used easily by health professionals such as health visitors, midwives and GPs. However, the EPDS is not intended to replace clinical judgment.

> The EPDS should be used as an adjunct to, not a replacement for, clinical judgment.
>
> *(Holden, 1994, p. 126)*

Although the EPDS is generally viewed as a positive development and a useful screening tool, there are some reservations with its use. Elliot (1994) writes that the problem may not necessarily be with the questionnaire itself, but with the expectations of what it can be reasonably expected to achieve. Elliot states that the EPDS is often used in a way that is unfocused in its intent:

> The EPDS is often used without any clear ideas to what it is being used for, so inappropriate decisions are made on administration and scoring. It is necessary to be clear about differences between the general population and the population being tested, and between those who should be referred on and those who should not.
>
> *(Elliot, 1994, p. 22)*

Elliot maintains that as referral mechanisms are not defined, and because the EPDS increases the detection rate, this can generate stress in professionals who are scoring the questionnaire. Part of this stress may relate to the increased workload of professionals such as health visitors, who already have considerable workloads and may have difficulty following up and referring women with high scores.

Women have expressed fears of being 'watched over' and are reluctant to complete the questionnaire (Comport, 1987). This may lead to the temptation either to resist filling in the questionnaire or to falsify the answers to avoid being labelled as mentally ill or being identified as an inadequate mother. Another potential problem with the use of the EPDS is that it may represent just another form to complete. During pregnancy, it is now fairly common for women to be bombarded by evaluation forms, paperwork and questionnaires as health service providers seek to gain more information about audit and quality of service provision. Another questionnaire may in this light be just another irritating piece of paper in a long line of many such surveys.

Other potential disadvantages of using a questionnaire screening process is that it might replace the importance of professionals getting to know their clients and developing supportive relationships. However, as has already been established, without the use of such a device the detection rate does not reflect the incidence of distress or depression. Ideally, it should be used as a supportive tool, so that screening does not diagnose yet helps to heighten professional awareness and detection whilst not replacing other communication skills of health professionals.

Holden (1994) maintains that the deployment of the EPDS gives women permission to speak and professionals permission to listen. What it probably does is to ensure that time is taken to reflect upon emotional changes, with it acting as a springboard to explore emotional reactions to motherhood. It is also felt that using the EPDS in clinical practice encourages women to seek help from other people as opposed to perhaps struggling on with an unacknowledged problem. Holden also believes that the EPDS can alter women's perceptions of what is available to them and become more aware of what health professionals are actually able to offer in terms of emotional support.

One of the definite advantages of the EPDS in the present climate of budget management, prioritising of service provision, audit and quality control is that it can be used as tool for change. By producing documentable evidence of the incidence rate and proof for need of service provision, the EPDS can be used as a tool to convince health service managers that there is a case to provide more efficient and effective services.

As the EPDS is suitable to be used by different types of health professionals, it is possible that it may encourage interdisciplinary liaison. However, two of the problems that women with emotional problems, distress or depression face concerns which professional group is the provider of care and how this care is then funded. Obstetric care, psychiatric care and health visitor care, for example, all come under separate trust status in many areas, and many more

GPs are moving towards fund holder status. It is possible to argue that this may present a conflict in care priorities and could result in a deficit of care provision for women who need support with a multifocused approach.

The EPDS was designed to be used at 6 weeks postpartum, and Holden (1994) believes that this gives the opportunity for early preventive and intervention measures. However, as the EPDS has proved to be an effective and efficient screening tool, it has also been introduced for use antenatally. Previous research (for example, Green and Murray, 1994), has shown that antenatal symptoms correlate closely with postnatal symptoms. Cox (1994) writes that as development and exploration of the EPDS continues it may be pertinent to change its name to the Edinburgh Perinatal Depression Scale or the Edinburgh Depression Scale. There may also be the possibility of using the EPDS to identify depressed fathers.

However, Painter (1995) has identified problems following the use of the EPDS. In a health visitor project, the value of the EPDS in helping to identify postnatal depression and the value of early health visitor intervention were evaluated. What Painter found was that the EPDS was a useful tool for health visitor use, as, except in cases of demanding and heavy caseloads, the EPDS can realistically be incorporated into an existing health service. In terms of service provision, utilising the EPDS enabled the health visitors to identify a lack of provision for clients' needs, particularly in terms of the number of community psychiatric nurses and counsellors from the National Childbirth Trust. However, this did result in liaison with mental health teams and a clearer focus upon how to evolve shared roles.

Problems were, however, identified by some of the health visitors who participated in the scheme:

> One health visitor was unable to use the EPDS on the majority of her clients due to heavy caseload demands. One health visitor raised the issue that GP fundholders may be unwilling to accept the use of EPDS, with the associated possibility of increased home visiting an higher demands on budgets.
>
> *(Painter, 1995, p. 40)*

Two of the health visitors in the scheme who were attached to fund holding GPs felt that the fund holding practice was unlikely to see the implementation of EPDS use as a workload priority. This, however, reflects not upon the validity of the EPDS as a screening tool, but more on present health-care priorities and economics.

The use of screening questionnaires is not new and there is continuing research into this area. For example, the CASE (Cognitive Adaptation to Stressful Events Scale) Instrument has been used to test women's cognitive adaptation to stressful events during pregnancy and the postpartum period (Affonso et al., 1994). The underlying theoretical base of CASE is conceived around Taylor's theory of cognitive adaption to threatening events (1983). Affonso et al.'s research indicated that CASE has potential in clinical screening as it looks at dysfunctional thought patterns and can be used to implement early preventive measures. The research, which is American based, does not, however, indicate whether it would be as user friendly for UK health professionals as the EPDS appears to be.

McClarey and Stokoe (1995) have reported on multidisciplinary innovations in the treatment and detection of postnatal depression.

> Health visitors in Oxford city had been identifying postnatal depression in their annual assessment of factors affecting health. However this view was mainly based upon perceptions; consequently the range of responses concerning the incidence of postnatal illness in health visitor caseloads was largely inaccurate.
>
> *(McClarey and Stokoe, 1995, p. 141)*

Previous attempts at using the EPDS were not satisfactory, and health professionals remained concerned over the lack of consensus over the management of postnatal depression.

The Oxford strategy principally aimed to improve the detection rates and reduce the effects by screening women using the EPDS. This would be achieved by training health visitors fully to utilise their skills and finally to raise the profile of postnatal depression to benefit health professionals and women.

The steering group for initiation of the Oxford strategy consisted of the senior nurse for health visiting, a senior midwife, a community psychiatric nurse, a member of the health promotion unit, a GP, a purchaser, a consultant psychologist and a register in obstetric liaison psychiatry.

The benefits and positive outcomes from this research showed through its collaborative nature. McClarey and Stokoe (1995) identified the outcomes as follows. The strategy was developed to be client centered and, in collaboration, this was enhanced by flexibility in professional boundaries. Having used a assessment system that could be validated, outcomes can then be identified and quantified. The strategy was devised to utilise working practices of health visitors, midwives and GPs. Finally, the strategy is structured to allow dynamic development. McClarey and Stokoe believe that the Oxford city strategy could act as a blueprint for the success of other multi-disciplinary schemes across the country.

Health professionals also have a role to play in helping to initiate, and act as facilitators in, peer group support groups. This allows a mingling of principles. The idea is that of professional guidance in group formation, structure and identification, followed by giving space to women to explore their own needs and feelings. This leads on to the role of voluntary groups, self-directed peer groups and structured groups.

Voluntary and peer support

Cutrona and Troutman (1986) wrote that women who had other women to rely upon had more confidence in their abilities as mothers and that this confidence acted as an effective deterrent to depression.

In acting as facilitators to peer support groups, health professionals can access premises, help with provision of facilities such as crèches and coordinate initial meetings. Gordon et al. (1995) hoped to facilitate a group similar to that established in Nottingham (Rowe, 1993), enabling women to define their own needs, and be active in the group dynamic process.

The group is structured in that different subjects are approached each week. Subjects have included stress management, parenting and childhood illnesses. Having the group setting gives women the opportunity to share their experiences, thus providing each other with support:

> For many mothers these groups provided the only opportunity in their day-to-day lives where they feel free to express secret feelings and concerns, many said they were relieved at not having to keep these bottled up.
>
> *(Gordon* et al.*, 1995, p. 156)*

Similar support groups have been formed, for example the Maidenhead Postnatal Help Group was established in 1986 (Jones et al., 1995). This was a collaboration between local health visitors and the local National Childbirth Trust. Again, rates of referral have increased since the introduction of the EPDS.

> The Maidenhead postnatal support group does not claim to cure illness, nor even to help alleviate its symptoms. But it does help in getting the client through the dreadful period of the illness by assuring sympathy and support within a network of fellow sufferers.
>
> *(Jones* et al., 1995, p. 155)*

Eastwood (1995) has identified the following advantages of peer support groups:

- The women in the group realised for the first time that they were not alone, that other women had had similar experiences.
- The sharing of experiences gave the women insight into different perspectives.
- The group was confidential, and this facilitated an atmosphere of openness and trust.
- Increased knowledge about postnatal depression enabled the women to realise that what they felt was normal.
- There was an increase in the self-esteem of the women.

Again, women stated that partners should become more involved in group activities so that they could gain insights into the effects of childbirth and childrearing and thus have more insight into the women's experiences. This could take the form of men-only groups. There are many schemes running across the country that involve peer group support and are coordinated by health professionals; however, there is no consistent access across the country, and many women do not have this style of support available to them.

Other support groups are run on a voluntary basis, and although the groups may have national status, such as the National Childbirth Trust, Newpin and Homestart, it very much depends upon the locality as to what is available (see Appendix IV for a list of national support agencies that may offer either a centralised or a local service). Types of support concentrated on so far have been professional help and peer group support with an emphasis on stress management, counselling, confidence building and group dynamics. However, other different types of support are also available in different areas.

May (1995) writes about an initiative in Dundee involving exercise and relaxation sessions. This initiative was originally started by a health visitor concerned with the high levels of depression within her caseload. May found that the exercise and relaxation promoted feelings of wellbeing, but, importantly, the group dynamics again provided peer group support. Other support groups involve a variety of activities such as yoga, massage, aromatherapy and drama therapy. Again, the availability of these therapies depends upon locality and the distribution of voluntary groups.

Preventive measures

If treatment is one approach to the problem of postnatal depression and maternal distress, prevention of the problem is an earlier starting point. For some women, depression will occur regardless of what happens, but preventive measures could lessen the severity of the problem, alert women to the access to support and potentially alert health professionals to women who are likely to develop problems.

Clements (1995) looked at the validity of introducing 'listening visits' antenatally, targeting in particular women with low emotional wellbeing. Clements found that this was potentially effective in preventing postnatal depression but that more research was required. Midwives in some areas are already incorporating open discussion and psychological perspectives in client interaction. This can take place as part of the initial booking visit, which is in some areas now more client focused, with visits taking place in the home environment, and less rigid in format. The concept is of the named midwife and midwifery caseloads. Clements feels that a structured approach to identifying women with a potential to develop problems would focus the listening visits in a time-structured way. This could be achieved by the use of the EPDS.

Appleby et al. (1989) looked at establishing a psychiatric liaison service within an obstetric unit. The aim of this service was antenatally to predict women at risk of postnatal depression and then to follow them up through pregnancy and in the postpartum period. Appleby et al. found that there was a large demand for the liaison service, although this did not always develop from the initial aims of the service. Appleby et al. concluded that the demands of such a service would imply expanding available resources:

It is indisputable that the psychiatric complications of pregnancy are common, distressing and potentially serious, and it follows that a liaison service should be expanded in accordance with the magnitude of the problems it addresses. Only a properly resourced service can evaluate and improve its methods and management towards both efficient prediction of risk and more effective treatment.

(Appleby et al., 1989, p. 510)

Elliot et al. (1988) looked at the use of parenting groups focusing parenting skills, relationships and social support. Again, this proved effective for prevention of postnatal depression in a group of women already identified as vulnerable. This approach could be effectively

178

utilised for use in parentcraft groups in general, and again this is another area where parentcraft educators are responding to the needs of women rather than their own preordained structure. The use of parentcraft is a useful preventive measure. However, its drawback as a broad-spectrum measure is that not all women attend parentcraft sessions, so many women may not benefit from this.

The concept of debriefing post-delivery may also have a significant impact on the development of depression and distress. The basic principle of debriefing is that each individual woman is given the opportunity to discuss and go through the events of her labour and delivery. It is hoped that this debriefing would prevent the development of emotional difficulties (Charles and Curtis, 1994). There is currently a debate over when it is most appropriate to use debriefing and who is the most appropriate person to carry it out. Relf and Alexander (1994) noted that midwives already use debriefing in an informal capacity in varying degrees. Critical incident stress debriefing takes place roughly 24–48 hours post-traumatic experience. In childbirth, this could be appropriate given the early discharge rates from hospital and the deployment of staff. It could depend on who the woman had the best relationship with. However, in instances where the birth was traumatised by inadequate staff, the woman may find it difficult to talk with the midwives involved in that experience. In an integrated midwifery service, where the principle of midwifery caseloads predominates, a midwife would ideally know her clients antenatally, offer interpartum care and continue with her care postnatally. This would then enable the woman and the midwife to use the principles of both listening visits and debriefing at a mutually convenient time. The personal experience of the authors has found that 28-day follow-up visits with clients to be a valuable addition to clinic practice. However, if large caseloads are involved, it can be a time-consuming activity that interferes with other clinical demands. To fully incorporate psychologically orientated visits into clinical practice, health professionals need to be adequately resourced.

If health professionals are going to seriously take on board prevention of maternal distress and postnatal depression, they need to be adequately prepared through changes in course content coupled with an emphasis in post-qualification training. Midwives have always been required to maintain their qualification by regular updating, and the English National Board (ENB) is increasingly widening the scope of its validation of recognised study days. For example, in 1995 the annual conference of the Society for Reproductive and Infant Psychology received ENB validation, enabling midwives to count attendance as validated study days. The course contents of educational programmes now include components on women and health, communication and counselling skills, and psychological aspects of health.

The Expert Maternity Group's report (1993) clearly stated what women have demanded of the maternity services:

> Above all, women and their partners are seeking a service that is respectful, personalized and kind, which gives them control and makes them feel comfortable in the sense of being at ease in the environment of childbirth and having confidence in their care.
>
> *(Department of Health, 1993, Foreword)*

It is hoped that the changes envisaged and legislated for in *Changing Childbirth* (see Appendix I) will allow women to make their own choices, letting them take more control, as we have previously identified that lack of control is problematic for women in childbirth. Riley (1995) has also recommended that changes are made to the training of health professionals to facilitate prevention, detection and treatment of postnatal depression and maternal distress.

It is hoped that the measures identified in this chapter will, with increased awareness, become available on a national basis for women, thus helping to decrease levels of depression and distress through preventive measures and improved education of health professionals. These actions should prepare women more realistically for the reality of childbirth and make them aware of what help is available. When depression and distress do occur, improved service provision and support should aid early detection and treatment. Increased public awareness of the psychological minefields associated with childbirth might remove some of the feelings of inadequacy that affect many distressed women, and improve self-help seeking actions. Having a child is supposed to be a positive experience; for many women, it is a hidden nightmare laden with mental torment and self-torture. The aim of health professionals and carers should be to prevent maternal distress and depression as much as possible and to be as supportive as possible when difficulties do arise:

> I have one thirteen year old son, physically I recovered quickly, mentally I am so scarred by that experience that I vowed I would never put myself through that again. It's not fair on me, my husband, my family and my son.
>
> *(Personal communication to authors)*

References

Affonso, D. D., Mayberry, L. T., Lovett, S. and Paul, S. (1994) 'Cognitive Adaptation to Stressful Events during Pregnancy and Post Partum: Development and Testing of the CASE Instrument.' *Nursing Research* **43**(6): 338–43.

Appleby, L., Fox, H., Shaw, M. and Kumar, R. (1989) 'The Psychiatrist in the Obstetric Unit: Establishing a Liaison Service.' *British Journal of Psychiatry* **154**: 510–15.

Ashurst, P. and Hall, Z. (1989) *Understanding Women in Distress* (London: Tavistock/Routledge).

Beck, A. T., Ward, C. H. and Mendelsohn, M. (1961) 'An Inventory for Measuring Depression.' *Archives of General Psychiatry* **4**: 53–63.

Bedford, A. and Foulds, G. (1978) *Delusions Symptoms States: States of Anxiety and Depression* (Windsor: National Foundation for Educational Research).

Charles, J. and Curtis, L. (1994) 'Birth Afterthoughts – a Listening and Information Service.' *British Journal of Midwifery* **2**: 331–4.

Clements, S. (1995) 'Listening Visits' in 'Pregnancy: A Strategy for Preventing Postnatal Depression?' *Midwifery* **11**: 75–80.

Comport, M. (1987) *Towards Happy Motherhood: Understanding Postnatal Depression* (London: Corgi).

Cox, J. L. (1986) *Postnatal Depression* (London: Churchill Livingstone).

Cox,. J. L., Holden, J. M., Sagovsky, K. (1987) 'Detection of Postnatal Depression: Development of the 10 Item EPDS.' *British Journal of Psychiatry* **150**: 782–6.

Cox, J. L., Gerrard, J., Cookson, D. and Jones J. M. (1993) 'Development and Audit of Charles Street Parent and Baby Day Unit, Stoke on Trent.' *Psychiatric Bulletin* **17**: 711–13.

Cutrona, C. E. and Troutman, B. R. (1986), 'Social Support, Infant Temperament and Parenting Self Efficiency: A Medicational Model of Post Partum Depression.' *Child Development* **57**: 1507–18.

Department of Health (1993) *Changing Childbirth.* The Report of the Expert Maternity Group. (London: HMSO).

Department of Health (1993) *The Health of the Nation: Key Area Handbook on Mental Illness* (London: HMSO).

Eastwood, P. (1995) 'Promoting Peer Group Support with Postnatally Depressed Women.' *Health Visitor* **68**(4): 148–50.

Elliot, S. A. (1994) 'Uses and Misuses of the EPDS in Primary Care: A Comparison of Models Developed in Health Visiting.' In Cox, J. L. and Holden, J. (eds) *Perinatal Psychiatry* (London: Gaskell).

Elliot, S. A., Sanjack, M. and Leverton, T. J. (1988), 'Parent's Groups in Pregnancy: A Preventative Intervention for Postnatal Depression?' In Gottleib, B. J. (ed.) *Marshaling Social Support* (California: Sage).

Goldberg, D. P. (1972) *The Detection of Psychiatric Illness by Questionnaires* (Oxford: Oxford University Press).

Gordon, J., Robertson, R. and Swan, M. (1995) '"Babies Don't Come with a Set of Instructions": Running Support Groups for Mothers.' *Health Visitor* **68**(4): 155–6.

Green, J. M. and Murray, D. (1994) 'The Use of the EPDS in Research to Explore the Relationship between Antenatal and Postnatal Dysphoria.' In Cox, J. L. and Holden, J. (eds) *Perinatal Psychiatry* (London: Gaskell).

Holden, J. M. (1994) 'Using the Edinburgh Postnatal Depression Scale in Clinical Practice.' In Cox, J. L. and Holden, J. M. (eds) *Perinatal Psychiatry: Use and Misuse of the EPDS* (London: Gaskell).

Jones, A., Watts, T. and Romain, S. (1995) 'Facilitating Peer Group Support.' *Health Visitor* **68**(4): 153.

Lindsay, J. S. B. and Pollard, D. E. (1978) 'Mothers and Children in Hospital.' *Australia and New Zealand Journal of Psychiatry* **12**: 245–53.

May, A. (1995), 'Using Exercise to Tackle Postnatal Depression.' *Health Visitor* **68**(4): 146–7.

McClarey, M. and Stokoe, B. (1995) 'A Multi-disciplinary Approach to Postnatal Depression.' *Health Visitor* **68**(4): 141–4.

McIntosh, J. (1993) 'Post Partum Depression: Women's Help Seeking Behaviour and Perceptions of Cause.' *Journal of Advanced Nursing* **18**:178–84.

Oates, M. (1988) 'The Development of an Integrated Community Orientated Service for Severe Postnatal Depression.' In Kumar, R. and Brockington, I. F. (eds) *Motherhood and Mental Illness 2* (London: Wright).

Painter, A. (1995) 'Health Visitor Identification of Postnatal Depression.' *Health Visitor* **68**(4): 138–40.

Prettyman, R. J. and Friedman, T. (1991) 'Care of women with Puerperal Psychiatric Disorders in England and Wales.' *British Medical Journal* **302**:1245–6.

Relf, K. and Alexander, J. (1994) 'Born Under Stress.' *Nursing Times* **90**(12): 29–30.

Riley, D. (1995) *Perinatal Mental Health* (Oxford: Radcliffe Medical Press).

Rowe, A. (1993) 'Cope Street Revisited.' *Health Visitor* **66**(10): 358–9.

Taylor, A., Adams, D. and Glover, V. (1994) 'Postnatal Depression: Identification, Risks Factors and Effects.' *British Journal of Midwifery* **2**(6): 253–7.

Taylor, S. (1983) 'A Theory of Cognitive Adaptation.' *American Psychologist* **38**: 1161–73.

Winterton Report (1992) *Health Committee Second Report on the Maternity Services*, vol. 1 (London: HMSO).

APPENDICES

Indicators of Success in
Changing Childbirth

The following should be achieved within 5 years.

1. All women to carry their own notes
2. Every woman to have a 'named midwife'
3. At least 30% of women should have a midwife as the lead professional
4. Every woman to know the lead professional who plans and provides her care
5. 75% of women should know the person who cares for them during their delivery
6. Midwives should have direct access to some beds in all maternity units
7. 30% of women delivered in a maternity unit should be under the management of a midwife
8. Total number of antenatal visits for women with uncomplicated pregnancies should have been reviewed in the light of available evidence and the RCOG guidelines
9. Front line ambulances to have a paramedic able to support the midwife who needs to transfer a woman to hospital in an emergency
10. All women to have access to information about the services available in their locality

Source: Department of Health (1993) Changing Childbirth. The Report of the Expert Maternity Group. *(London: HMSO).*

The Edinburgh Postnatal Depression Scale

Today's date: _____   Baby's age: _____

Baby's date of birth: _____   Birth weight: _____

Triplets/Twins/Single   Male/Female

Mother's age: _____

Number of other children: 0 1 2 3 4 5 5+

How are you feeling?

As you have recently had a baby, we would like to know how you are feeling now. Please <u>underline</u> the answer which comes closest to how you have felt in the past 7 days, not just how you feel today.

Here is an example, already completed.

I have felt happy:

> Yes, most of the time
>
> <u>Yes, some of the time</u>
>
> No, not very often
>
> No, not at all

This would mean: 'I have felt happy some of the time' during the past week. Please complete the other questions in the same way.

The Edinburgh Postnatal Depression Scale

IN THE PAST SEVEN DAYS	Score

1. I have been unable to laugh and see the funny side of things:

As much as I always could	0
Not quite as much now	1
Definitely not so much now	2
Not at all	3

2. I have looked forward with enjoyment to things:

As much as I ever did	0
Rather less than I used to	1
Definitely less than I used to	2
Hardly at all	3

3. I have blamed myself unnecessarily when things went wrong:

Yes, most of the time	0
Yes, some of the time	1
Not very often	2
No, never	3

4. I have felt worried and anxious for no good reason:

No, not at all	0
Hardly ever	1
Yes, sometimes	2
Yes, very often	3

5. I have felt scared or panicky for no very good reason:

Yes, quite a lot	0
Yes, sometimes	1
No, not much	2
No, not at all	3

6. Things have been getting on top of me:

Yes, most of the time I haven't been able to cope at all	0
Yes, sometimes I haven't been coping as well as usual	1
No, most of the time I have coped quite well	2
No, I have been coping as well as ever	3

7. I have been so unhappy that I have difficulty sleeping:

Yes, most of the time	0
Yes, sometimes	.1
Not very often	2
No, not at all	3

8. I have felt sad or miserable:

Yes, most of the time	0
Yes, quite often	1
Not very often	2
No, not at all	3

9. I have been so unhappy that I have been crying:

Yes, most of the time	0
Yes, quite often	1
Only occasionally	2
No, never	3

10. The thought of harming myself has occurred to me:

Yes, quite often	0
Sometimes	1
Hardly ever	2
Never	3

Taken from Cox, J. L., Holden, J. M. and Sagovsky, R. (1987) 'Detection of Postnatal Depression: Development of the 10 Item Edinburgh Postnatal Depression Scale.' British Journal of Psychiatry *130*: 782–8. Reproduced by kind permission of the Royal College of Psychiatrists.

Probable and Potential Interventions During Labour and Childbirth

Artificial rupture of membranes

Example of some indications

In some units, this still remains a policy. Membranes are routinely ruptured at 3–4 cm cervical dilatation. Membranes may be ruptured as part of induction and augmentation of labour, in order to site fetal scalp electrodes, to assess fetal distress (determine whether meconium is present), to accelerate labour or to perform fetal blood sampling.

Potential problems

Can cause fetal distress: the pressure of contractions will be directly onto the fetus.

Contractions usually become more painful and there is an increased use of pharmacological analgesia.

The fetus is no longer protected by a bag of sterile fluid.

It limits the length of labour before further interventions are required to complete the process.

Caesarean section

Example of some indications

Planned: predisposing obstetric, medical or fetal reasons.

Emergency: possibly life-threatening reasons, for example cord prolapse or abruption. Alternatively, those that are unplanned but with less immediate urgency. The woman will also be catheterised, and have an intravenous infusion and a partial shave of pubic hair.

Potential problems

If a general anaesthetic is used, the woman may feel ill while recovering and will not see her baby immediately at birth.

There may be problems relating to urinary retention, infection or trauma.

Pain is associated with the major abdominal surgery.

Limited mobility may make feeding and care of the baby more difficult.

It can result in psychological distress.

It may be associated with distorted body image.

Continuous fetal monitoring

Example of some indications

External: Many units consider this to be a standard procedure. Contractions are usually also measured. The purpose is to observe the wellbeing or distress of the fetus.

Potential problems

Mobility is limited and abdominal belts may be uncomfortable. The machine requires regular servicing to ensure that the information given is accurate and leads and belts require (but do not always receive) cleaning between deliveries. Monitoring can lead to further intervention.

Entonox

Example of some indications

Analgesia.

Potential problems

Not always effective and is associated with nausea and feelings of lack of control in some women. May cause feelings of claustrophobia, and the mouthpiece and mask can cause a dry mouth.

Epidural anaesthesia

Examples of some indications

To reduce the experience of pain or to reduce blood pressure in women with hypertensive diseases of pregnancy.

Potential problems

Mobility reduction. Intravenous therapy will be required, and the woman is usually subjected to continuous fetal and contraction monitoring. Some women may experience difficulty in passing urine and may require temporary catheterisation – a potential source of infection. If not managed properly, an epidural may increase the risk of an instrumental delivery and associated episiotomy. Postural problems may lead to backache.

Episiotomy

Example of some indications

To ease the birth of the baby. It is used in most instrumental deliveries and when fetal distress is present at the end of the second stage of labour. Is also employed where extensive perineal scarring is present or female genital mutilation has occurred.

Potential problems

The local anaesthetic may not be active prior to the cut. Blunt scissors may make the incision difficult to perform. A painful perineum may cause difficulties with feeding the baby, particularly so with breastfeeding. Stitches may be uncomfortable and may become infected and break down. Sexual intercourse may be painful for many months post-birth, and disturbance of body image may be present.

Fetal blood sampling

Example of some indications

To assess fetal wellbeing by measuring the pH of fetal blood. It involves lithotomy or the left lateral position. A hollow metal tube is introduced into the vagina to visualise the fetal presenting part. A small sample of blood is obtained and the information obtained allows more accurate decisions about further interventions.

Potential problems

Invasive, uncomfortable and, in certain instances, painful. It involves vaginal examination and, if necessary, artificially rupturing the membranes. If meconium is present and not adequately cleaned from the fetal presenting part, a false reading may be obtained.

Fetal scalp electrode

Example of some indications

It is sometimes used routinely, or used when external monitoring is not considered to be efficient.

Potential problems

It is invasive and involves artificially rupturing the membranes and performing a vaginal examination. It can be uncomfortable, limits mobility and is associated with a high risk of further interventions. It is a potential source of infection.

Forceps delivery

Examples of some indicators

It is used in incidences of fetal distress in the second stage of labour, for maternal exhaustion or where prolonged pushing is counter-indicated. It is also employed for slow progress in the second stage of labour, to rotate fetal head if the position is not favourable, and sometimes for caesarean sections and for the head in a breech birth.

Potential problems

Women are usually in the lithotomy position and catheterised. Forceps deliveries are usually accompanied by episiotomies. They cause some women psychological distress, and the fetus may suffer bruising to the head and temporary cerebral irritation.

Intravenous cannulae

Examples of some indications

These are given to women suspected of needing intravenous therapy, for example in induction of labour. Some units extend this to women who have previously undergone a caesarean section.

Potential problems

There can be discomfort and pain at the site. Their presence may increase the chance of further intervention. They may limit mobility (depending upon site) and are a potential source of infection/inflammation.

Intravenous infusions

Example of some indications

These are used for induction/augmentation of labour, when an epidural is in situ, for an underlying medical condition, in the prevention of premature labour and in caesarean sections.

Potential problems

These are painful to have sited and mobility is limited. They may need to remain in situ post-delivery (depending on the reason for their being sited initially) and can cause local infection.

Pethidine

Example of some indications

Analgesia.

Potential problems

Pethidine is only effective in approximately 50 per cent of women. Once given, it may cause side-effects, for example nausea, dizziness and feelings of loss of control. Pethidine needs to be given approximately 4 hours before delivery, which is not easy to predict. It affects the fetus and may interfere with suckling reflex and inhibit efficient feeding.

Speculum

Example of some indications

Examination using a speculum may be carried out to determine whether the membranes have ruptured when no contractions are present, to visualise the cervix to determine whether labour is premature or whether it is source of bleeding. It is also conducted to perform a high vaginal swab.

Potential problems

This can be uncomfortable or painful if not done carefully, and can be embarrassing.

Suturing

Example of some indications

Repair of tears to perineum, labia, clitoris, urethra and rectum; also for repair of an episiotomy.

Potential problems

It may be painful due to inadequate anaesthesia. There may be formation of scar tissue and a possibility of infection. Postural problems may lead to infant feeding difficulties, and there is a potential problem with micturation and defecation depending on the suture site. Sexual intercourse may be painful and disturbance of body image may occur.

Urinary catheterisation

Examples of some indications

This is carried out to empty a full bladder if the woman is unable to micturate (a temporary catheter). Its use is more likely if the woman has had an epidural. Catheterisation may occur if urine output needs to be closely monitored or if there is a delay (or problems) in the third stage of labour, and also prior to caesarean section and instrumental delivery.

Potential problems

It may contribute to bladder dysfunction. There is an increased risk of urinary tract infection, and it can cause urethral trauma if carried out incorrectly.

Vaginal examination

Example of some indications

Every woman has a vaginal examination to establish progress and the stage of labour, and to determine fetal position and descent. Examinations take place, on average, every 4 hours but may be conducted more frequently.

Potential problems

These may be experienced as invasive and/or embarrassing. The experience may be associated with discomfort or pain. They are a potential source of infection.

Ventouse delivery

Example of some indications

Ventouse delivery is used in incidences of fetal distress in the second stage of labour, for maternal exhaustion, where prolonged pushing is contraindicated and for slow progress during the second stage of labour.

Potential problems

Women are usually in the lithotomy position and catheterised. They are usually given an episiotomy. Ventouse delivery can cause the woman psychological distress. The fetus may have bruising on its head and temporary cerebral irritation.

Appendix IV

Organisations that offer help to mothers experiencing depression and other forms of postnatal distress

Action for Victims of Medical Accidents (AVMA)
Bank Chambers
Forest Hill
London SE23 3TP

Tel: 0181-291 2793

AVMA helps on a personal basis people who have been, or think they have been, victims of a medical accident.

Asian Family Counselling Service
74 The Avenue
London W13 8LB

Tel: 0181-997 5749

Assists families with marital problems and offers counselling.

Association of Community Health Councils for England and Wales
30 Drayton Park
London N5 1PB

Tel: 0171-609 8405

Provides information service on consumer rights. Contact the local Community Health Council via the local telephone dsirectory.

Association for Post Natal Illness (APNI)
25 Jerdan Place
London SW6 1BE

Tel: 0171-386 0868
(Mon–Fri 10.00 am – 5.00 pm)

Offers telephone support and advice by a network of volunteers who

have themselves suffered postnatal depression. For information packs, please send a size A5 SAE.

Association of Radical Midwives (ARM)
62 Greetby Hill
Ormskirk
Lancashire L39 2DT

Tel: 01695 572776

Support group for midwives and mothers, campaigning to enhance the choices of childbirth for women. Please send SAE with written enquiries.

Bliss – Baby Life Support Systems
17–21 Emerald Street
London WC1N 3QL

Tel: 0171-831 9393/8996

Raises funds for SCBUs and helps to provide vital equipment and training for doctors and nurses in fast-developing techniques. Blisslink offers a support network for parents, helping them cope with the inevitable distress. There is a newsletter, leaflets and telephone support.

Body Positive
51B Philbeach Gardens
London SW5 9EB

Head Office Tel: 0171-835 1045
Helpline: 0171-373 9124 (Mon–Fri 7 pm – 10 pm;
Sat –Sun 4 pm – 10 pm)

Support and information advice regarding HIV/AIDS.

British Association for Counselling
1 Regent Place
Rugby CV21 2PJ

Tel: 01788 550899

Directory of qualified counsellors. Please write sending an SAE. A list of counsellors will be forwarded by return of post

Caesarean Support Group
Alexandra House
Oldham Terrace
London W3 6NH

Tel: 0181-992 8637

Offers information and support.

Caesarean Support Network
c/o 55 Coil Drive
Douglas
Isle of Man IM2 2HF

Tel: 01624 661269

Offers support to women who will, who know they will, or who have had a caesarean and who want to have a normal birth in the future.

CARE
3 Alder Grove
Normanton
West Yorkshire WF6 1LF

Tel: 01924 894076

A self-help 'phone line', mainly for birth mothers, coping with adoption-related experiences, but anyone who has experience of adoption is welcome to contact.

CARE The Scottish Association for Care and Support After the Diagnosis of Fetal Abnormality
Griselda Gordon
Stair House Farm
Mauchline, Ayrshire KA3 5PS

Tel: 01292 591741

Self-help network – self-help after termination. Telephone befriending, and self-help during a subsequent pregnancy.

Central Office of Homestart UK
2 Salisbury Road
Leicester LE1 7QR

Tel: 0116 233 9955

Practical help and emotional support for mothers with at least one child under school age

Compassionate Friends
53 North Street
Bristol BS3 1EN

Helpline: 0117 9539 639

A nationwide organisation of bereaved parents offering friendship and understanding to other bereaved parents after the death of a son or daughter from any cause. Personal and group support. There is a quarterly newsletter, a postal library and a range of leaflets. Provides support for bereaved siblings and grandparents. Emphasis is on befriending rather than counselling.

CRUSE
Bereavement Care
126 Sheen Road
Richmond
Surrey TW9 1UR

Tel: 0181-940 4808

CRUSE bereavement line (0181-332 7227) provides a direct link with a counsellor Mon–Fri 9.30 am – 5 pm. Free help via local branches, which offer individual and group counselling. Social contacts and practical advice. Has a publications list and a newsletter.

CRY-SIS
B.M. CRY-SIS
London WC1N 3XX

Tel: 0171-404 5011
8.00 am to 11.00 pm every day of the year.

Mainly telephone support, a listening service run by people who have a crying child. Provides emotional support, advice and tips on coping with excessively crying, sleepless and demanding babies and children. Please send SAE when writing.

Exploring Parenthood
4 Ivory Place
22A Treadgold Street
London W11 4BP

Admin. Tel: 0181 960 1678
Advice Tel: 0171-221 6681

National telephone advice line. Various publications on all aspects of parenting, working with parents and also with professionals working with parents. Training packs for health and all other professionals. Moyenda Project working with African Caribbean and Asian families. 'Black Father's Talking' project, which supports black fathers.

Family CARE
21 Castle Street
Edinburgh EH2 3DN

Tel: 0131-225 6441

Adoption enquiry and counselling service. Provides a limited infertility counselling service.

Family Contact Line
30 Church Street
Altrincham
Cheshire WA14 4DW

Tel: 0161-941 4011/2

Confidential listening service, aiming to reduce stresses that lead

to child abuse. Counselling for adult survivors of child sex abuse, both male and female. Support for women suffering from postnatal depression. Counselling for various relationship problems. Affiliated to Parent-Line.

Foundation for the Study of Infant Deaths
14 Halkin Street
London SW1X 7DP

Tel: 0171-235 0965
24-hour cot death helpline: 0171-235 1721

The foundation funds research to find out why these tragedies occur and helps families devastated by cot death. Informs and educates health professionals and the public. Gives advice to parents on how they can reduce the risk of cot death.

Gingerbread
35 Wellington Street
London WC2E 7BN

Tel: 0171-240 0953

Association for one-parent families.

ISSUE (The National Fertility Association – England, Wales and Ireland)
509 Aldridge Road
Great Barr
Birmingham B44 8NA

Tel: 0121-344 4414

Self-help information and support for people with fertility problems.

LABS (The London Association of Bereavement Services)
London Voluntary Sector Resource Centre
356 Holloway Road
London N7 6PN

Tel: 0171-700 8134

Telephone helpline for bereaved people in Greater London. Referrals are to local service or to other organisations. In-service training for volunteers and professionals. Advice for those wishing to establish a service.

La Lèche League
BM3434
London WC1N 3XX

Tel: 0171-242 1278

Information and support on breastfeeding.

Marcé Society
c/o Dr T. Friedman
The Psychiatric Department
Leicester General Hospital
Gwendoline Road
Leicester LE5 4PW

Tel: 0131-317 3000 and 0116-249 0490

Professional body for anybody connected with the medical profession.

MAMA (Meet-a-Mum Association)
14 Willis Road
Croydon CRO 2XX

Tel: 0181-665 0357

Friendship and support on a mum-to-mum basis. Specific information and support for postnatal depression. Offers helpline numbers, open Mon–Fri, 6 pm – 11.00 pm and weekends 11.00 am to 8.00 pm.

Maternity Alliance
15 Brittannia Street
London WC1X 9JN

Tel: 0171-837 1265

Works to make life better for mothers, fathers and babies.

Maternity and Health Links
Old Co-op
42 Chelsea Road
Easton
Bristol BS5 6AF

Tel: 0117 955 8495

Support and English tuition to antenatal and postnatal non-English-speaking women. Interpreting and advocacy service.

Miscarriage Association
c/o Clayton Hospital
Northgate
Wakefield
West Yorkshire WF1 3JS

Tel: 01924 200799

Provides information and support for women who have suffered a miscarriage. Has a network of local contacts around the UK with women who can share their feelings. Also publishes information leaflets on aspects of miscarriage.

MIND (National Association for Mental Health)
Gransta House
15–19 Broadway
Stratford
London E15 4BQ

Tel: 0181-519 2122

Publishes various leaflets, including 'Understanding Post Natal Depression', 50p and an SAE to Publications Department of the above.

National Childbirth Trust (NCT)
Alexandra House
Oldham Terrace
London W3 6NH

Tel: 0181-992 8637

Offers information and support to parents.

National Council of Voluntary Child Care Organisations
Unit 4
Pride Court
80–82 White Lion Street
London N1 9PF

Tel: 0171-833 3319

Umbrella organisation for voluntary childcare organisations.

National Council for One Parent Families
255 Kentish Town Road
London NW5 2LX

Tel: 0171-267 1361

Enables lone parents to become financially independent. Referral service and return to work schemes. Advice on being single and pregnant.

Natural Parents Network
10 Alandale Crescent
Garforth
Leeds LS25 1DH

*Tel: 0113 286 8489
(Mon 9 am –1 pm, Tues–Thur 6 pm – 7 pm)*

Support for parents who have lost a child through adoption. Open Mon 9 am – 1 pm, Tue–Thur 6 pm – 7 pm.

NORCAP (National Organisation for the Counselling of Adoptees and Parents)
112 Church Road
Wheatley
Oxfordshire OX33 1LU

Tel: 01865 875000

Support for adult adoptees and birth and adoptive parents. Telephone counselling service. Search and research service. Liaison service; send an SAE when writing.

NSPCC (National Society for Prevention of Cruelty to Children)
National Centre
42 Curtain Road
London EC2A 3NH

Tel: 0171-825 2500

Will offer confidential support to parents.

Parent-Line National Office
Endway House
The Endway
Hadleigh
Essex SS7 2AN

*Helpline: 01702 559900
Admin. Tel: 01702 554782*

A helpline for parents under stress, for whatever reason.

Parent Network
44–46 Caversham Road
London NW5 2DS

Tel: 0171-485 8535

Parent LINK groups for parents are run by trained parents in their local communities at reasonable cost. The 13 sessions offer ideas for handling the daily ups and downs of family life in new ways to improve communication and to strengthen relationships.

Parents Anonoymous
6–7 Manor Gardens
London N7 6LA

Helpline: 0171-263 8918

A confidential listening service for parents to talk over any problem they, as a parent, may have.

Parents at Work
77 Holloway Road
London N7 8JZ

Helpline: 0171-700 5771
(Tue/Thur/Fri 11 am – 1 pm and
2 pm–4 pm)
Admin. Tel: 0171-700 5772

Practical advice on returning to
work after childbirth.

Positively Women
347–349 City Road
London EC1V 1LR

Tel: 0171-713 0444
Client Service Line: 0171-713 0222
12 pm to 2 pm daily

For women with HIV/related
conditions. Counselling advice on
pregnancy and children. African
Support Group Monday pm.

Post-Adoption Centre
5 Torriano Mews
Torriano Avenue
London NW5 2RZ

Tel: 0171-284 0555

Counselling for all people involved in
adoption.

**PROPES (Parents Recognition of
Paediatric Errors)**
Iatrongenic Centre
56 Southland Drives
West Cross
Swansea SA3 5RJ

Tel: 01792 403593

Support for parents by parents who
have faced or are facing or fighting
the wrong diagnosis of a child's
illness (or treatment at birth) and/or
death, by being labelled
'overanxious parents'.

RELATE
Marriage Guidance Council
Head Office
Herbert Grey College
Little Church Street
Rugby
Warwickshire CV21 3AP

Tel: 01788 573241

Support for people with relationship
problems.

**SANDS (Stillbirth and Neonatal
Death Society)**
28 Portland Place
London W1N 4DE

Tel: 0171-436 7940
Helpline: 0171-436 5881

Support for parents whose baby died
during late pregnancy or around the
time of birth. Support groups,
information support and literature.

**SATFA (Support Around
Termination for Abnormality)**
73 Charlotte Street
London W1P 1LB

Admin. Tel: 0171-631 0280
Parents Helpline: 0171-631 0285

Helping parents who discover that
their unborn baby is abnormal.
Works with professionals to improve
care.

Scottish Cot Death Trust
Royal Hospital for Sick Children
Yorkhill
Glasgow G3 8SJ

Tel: 0141-357 3946

Fund-raising for medical research
into cot death. Support of bereaved
parents. Education and information.

TAMBA (Twins and Multiple Births Association)
PO Box 30
Little Sutton
South Wirral L66 1TH

Tel: 0151-348 0020
(Mon–Fri 9 am – 1 pm)

Offers support for all the family. Specialist support groups. Bereavement, befriending, one-parent families, special needs, supertwins (triplets or more) and infertility support. Education and information, leaflets and literature. Local twin club.

Women's Aid Federation England
PO Box 391
Bristol BS99 7WS

Tel: 0117-963 3494

For women experiencing physical, emotional and sexual violence in the home. Local women's aid groups offering information, support, advice and refuge.

Women's Health Concern
PO Box 1629
London W8 6AU

Tel: 0171-938 3932

Information and advice for women with gynaecological and hormonal problems.

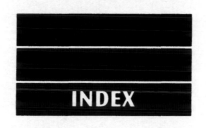

INDEX

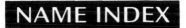

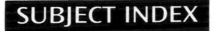

SUBJECT INDEX